THE CITY & GUILDS A-Z
HAIRDRESSING

About City & Guilds

City & Guilds is the UK's leading provider of vocational qualifications, offering over 500 awards across a wide range of industries and progressing from entry level to the highest levels of professional achievement. With over 8500 centres in 100 countries, City & Guilds is recognised by employers worldwide for providing qualifications that offer proof of the skills they need to get the job done.

Equal opportunities

City & Guilds fully supports the principle of equal opportunities and we are committed to satisfying this principle in all our activities and published material. A copy of our equal opportunities policy statement is available on the City & Guilds website.

Copyright

Designed and typeset by Select Typesetters Ltd
Printed in the UK by Swallowtail Print

Publications

For information about or to order City & Guilds support materials, contact 0844 534 0000 or centresupport@cityandguilds.com. You can find more information about the materials we have available at www.cityandguilds.com/publications.

Every effort has been made to ensure that the information contained in this publication is true and correct at the time of going to press. However, City & Guilds' products and services are subject to continuous development and improvement, and the right is reserved to change products and services from time to time. City & Guilds cannot accept liability for loss or damage arising from the use of information in this publication.

City & Guilds
1 Giltspur Street
London EC1A 9DD

T 0844 543 0033
www.cityandguilds.com
publishingfeedback@cityandguilds.com

CONTENTS

Acknowledgements   **4**

Introduction – how to use this book   **5**

The City & Guilds A–Z   **6**

ACKNOWLEDGEMENTS

Every effort has been made to acknowledge all copyright holders as below and the publishers will, if notified, correct any errors in future editions.

City & Guilds would like to sincerely thank the following:

For invaluable hairdressing expertise: Dawn Buttle and Diane Mitchell.

For providing pictures:

Adam Gault/Science Photo Library: p127; **Adam Sloan at Big Yin:** p113, 123; **Andover College:** pp8, 43, 46, 50, 50, 50, 96, 100, 102, 103, 118, 135; **Balmain:** pp25, 30, 49, 69, 95; **Banbury Postiche:** p59; **Barry Craig:** p131; **Cambridge Regional College:** pp25, 52, 68, 82, 83, 92, 105, 108; **Camera Press:** pp34, 36, 57, 95, 112, James Veysey 132; **Capital Hair & Beauty:** p116; **Carlton Group:** pp110, 128; **Central Sussex College:** p42; **Central Training Group:** pp10, 18, 31, 51, 96, 114, 130; **Cheynes Training:** pp14, 17, 17, 27, 38, 45, 59, 75, 95, 98, 117, 121, 133; **Clipso:** pp76, 128; **Clynol:** p9; **Conair:** p109; **Dani Free:** pp43, 60; **Denman Brush:** pp79, 84, 123, 126; **Desmond Murray:** pp14, 88, 129; **Ellisons:** p16; **Epping Forest College:** pp16, 19, 20, 20, 24, 27, 33, 43, 48, 49, 56, 57, 88, 93, 110, 116; **Errol Douglas MBE:** pp8, 42, 119, 125; **Essence PR:** p30; **Fotolia:** pp44, 53; **From Great Lengths:** pp33, 113; **Fudge:** p28; **GE Betterton:** p116; **Getty Images:** pp23, 31, 60, 87, 122, 132; **Goldwell:** pp7, 8, 11, 12, 18, 18, 30, 67, 70, 85, 90, 92, 99, 101, 103, 108, 115, 115, 118, 119, 127, 133; **Gorgeous PR:** p62; **Hair Tools:** p124; **Havering College:** pp11, 12, 31, 40, 44, 53, 71, 73, 84, 91, 97, 101, 103, 106, 110; **Hebe Salon:** p68; **Henley College, Coventry:** p78; **Hertford Regional College:** pp6, 14, 15, 16, 23, 24, 29, 36, 41, 44, 54, 54, 64, 65, 65, 76, 78, 79, 82, 84, 87, 87, 96, 99, 100, 115, 118; **Hob:** p42; **Hooker & Young:** p112; **India Today Group/Getty Images:** p96; **iStockphoto.com:** pp10, 11, 38, 117, 120; © alejandrophotography pp32, 106; © AllievanNiekerk p25; © AnajaCreatif pp30, 65; © AnthonyRosenberg p88; © aristotoo p20; © arlindo71 p91; © Arpad Benedek, Shelly Perry p55; © AYImages p74; © Cathy Britcliffe pp9, 39; © Danilin p81; © DinaTulchevska p27; © dissolvegirl p68; © DomenicoGelermo pp14, 95; © erierika p37; © espiegle p31; © Eulenblau p115; © Farina2000 p102; © fatihhoca pp29, 97; © Freegreen p13; © g_king p58; © Georgijevic p61; © greg801 p126; © herkisi p78; © Iconogenic pp10, 15, 24; © janulla p64; © jgroupp62; © Julia Shavchenko p52; © Kasiam p114; © labsas p33; © likim p73; © lissart pp106, 111; © luciancoman p36; © MariyaL p109; © mikdam pp48, 72; © Myroslav_Orshak p91; © Pete Fleming p22; © phakimata p88; © PIKSEL p11; © powerofforever pp38, 132; © pringletta pp34, 63, 108; © Quirex p60; © sdominick p62; © Stockphoto4u p82; © studio9 p12; © Sudo2 pp77, 94; © sweetlifephotos p47; © tderden p89; © xxmmxx p7; © yurok p74; **Jamie Stevens:** p15; Jeff Shanes: p27; **Joico:** p52; **KMS California:** pp53, 67, 77, 82, 123; **Kym Menzies-Foster; Photography by Andrew Buckle:** p80; **L'Oreal Professionnel:** p62; **Marino Lambrix/TONI&GUY:** p27; **Melissa Jenkins:** p6; **Michael Barnes:** p19; **Michelle Thompson at Francesco Group:** p63; **Mizani:** p39; **Mundo:** pp34, 42; **Oli Jones:** p66; **Patrick Cameron:** p23; **Rae Palmer:** p17; **Rainbow Room International:** p64; **Redken:** p121; **Richard Ward Hair & Metrospa:** pp17, 29, 36, 124; **Sanrizz:** pp55, 116; **Science Photo Library:** pp7, 9, 9, 13, 14, 20, 31, 54, 55, 64, 69, 73, 74, 82, 85, 112, 113, 116, 119, 122, 126, 130, 130, 131; **Shutterstock:** © Andriy Goncharenko p35; © conrado p100; © Photo_Creative p126; **Stephenson College:** p31; **The Academy, Enfield Training Services:** pp26, 59, 60, 61, 63, 86, 105; **The London College of Beauty Therapy:** pp32, 83, 91; **TIGI:** p28; **Tondeo:** p104; **TONI&GUY:** pp57, 70, 83, 92, 100, 105, 125; **Walsall College:** pp7, 12, 15, 20, 28, 38, 40, 41, 41, 46, 50, 57, 92, 93, 93, 98, 102, 107, 114, 121, 131, 132; **Wella:** pp30, 32, 72, 76, 93, 98, 98.

INTRODUCTION – HOW TO USE THIS BOOK

The City & Guilds A–Z contains the words you need to know if you're studying at level 1, 2 or 3, or if you're a qualified hairdresser. So if you haven't heard of a technical word before or need to refresh your memory, look it up in here.

Each word is followed by a phonetic respelling, so you know exactly how to pronounce it, as well as the actual definition, so you know exactly what it means.

The word

The phonetic respelling

The definition

Primary colours – PRIY-muh-ree KUH-luhz – Red, yellow and blue are the three colour pigments that cannot be made up from other colours. When mixing any two of these colours, secondary colours are produced, for example red plus yellow equals orange.

Processing time – PROH-sess-ing TIYM – The development time for a service.

Product build-up – PROD-uhkt BILD-up – When the hair has had excessive products applied, even though the hair is shampooed, the products still remain.

Productivity – prod-uhk-TIV-it-ee – This means the amount of work that you are getting done. If you work effectively, you will achieve high productivity.

Products – PROD-uhkts – Substances we use on our hair every day, eg shampoo, conditioner, styling gel and hairspray.

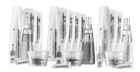

Prominent and protruding

Professional advice – pruh-FESH-uh-nuhl uhd-VYSS – Giving advice to a person based on your skills, knowledge and professional experiences.

Professional image – pruh-FESH-uh-nuhl IM-ij – Presenting yourself well in the salon, including following the rules of the dress code and using positive body language.

Professional indemnity insurance – pruh-FESH-uh-nuhl in-DEM-nit-ee in-SHOR-ruhnss – This will cover the salon against damages: for example, a customer might claim damages if their scalp is burned by incorrectly mixed chemicals.

Profit and loss – PROF-it uhnd LOSS – A financial statement that summarises the financial transactions for a business over a period in time.

Prominent and protruding – PROM-in-uhnt uhnd pruh-TROO-ding – Sticking out.

The City & Guilds A–Z Hairdressing 101

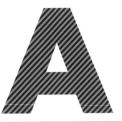

Abbreviation – uh-bree-vee-AY-shuhn – A shortened form of a word or phrase, normally used when making appointments, eg C/BD (cut and blow dry), S/S (shampoo and set), H/L (highlights) and P/W (perm winding).

Absorption – uhb-ZORP-shuhn – The capacity to soak up a substance.

Abundant – uh-BUN-duhnt – Great in amount or number.

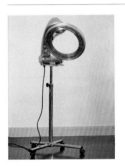

Accelerator – uhk-SEL-uh-ray-tuh – An appliance used to apply heat to the hair to speed up a service, eg steamers, rollerballs and climazones.

Access and egress – AK-sess uhnd EE-gress – All the routes into and out of the workplace. All corridors, doorways, steps and emergency exits, etc. must be kept free from obstructions and well maintained.

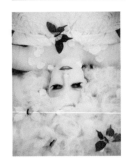

Accessory – uhk-SESS-uh-ree – An item, such as a fascinator, feathers or clips, used to complement a finished look.

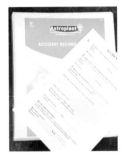

Accident book – AK-sid-uhnt BUUK – A book in the workplace where accidents are recorded; this is a requirement of health and safety law.

Acetone – ASS-i-tohn – A strong solvent found in some hair products.

Acid – ASS-id – Acids have a pH value below 7 and give off hydrogen ions in water.

Acid mantle – ASS-id MANTL – The acid mantle is a very fine, slightly acidic film on the surface of the skin acting as a barrier to bacteria, viruses and other potential contaminants that might penetrate the skin.

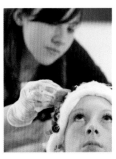

Acid perm
– ASS-id PURM
– Acid perms generally have a pH of 6–7 and are made up of a chemical ingredient called glyceryl monothioglycolate and an activator of thioglycolic acid.

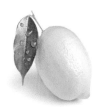

Acid rinse
– ASS-id RINSS
– Weak acids, such as lemon juice and vinegar diluted with water, can be applied to the hair after shampooing, making it shiny and closing the cuticle scales.

Acidic – uh-SID-ik – An acidic product will have a pH of less than 7.

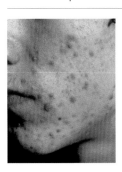

Acne vulgaris –
AK-nee vul-GAH-ris – A skin disorder which can be identified by spots and pustules, due to inflammation of the sebaceous glands.

Acrylic – uh-KRIL-ik – Made from synthetic (man-made) fibre.

Act – AKT – A law made by Parliament.

Action plan – AK-shuhn PLAN – Individuals can set personal goals that need to be achieved within a given timescale.

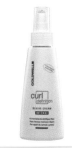

Activator –
AKT-iv-ay-tuh – A product used on wet hair to boost the curl in the hair.

Active listening – AK-tiv LISS-ning – Using techniques to show that you are paying close attention to what is being said by a client or colleague. For example, using eye contact, or repeating back what the person has said, to confirm understanding.

Acute dermatitis – uh-KYOOT dur-muh-TIY-tiss – Caused by exposure to an irritant and occurs almost immediately.

Adapting communication – uh-DAPT-ing kuh-myoo-ni-KAY-shuhn – You need to adapt your communication depending on the situation. Ways to do this are by using different tone and speed, using appropriate terminology, listening, and responding appropriately.

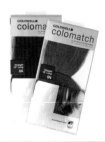

Added hair
– ADD-id HAIR –
Hair attached to the head or blended into the hair, for example hairpieces and extensions.

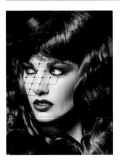

Additional media – uh-DISH-uh-nuhl MEE-dee-uh – Make-up, accessories, ornamentation, clothes, etc.

Additional services or products – uh-DISH-uh-nuhl SUR-viss-iz or PROD-uhkts – The additional services of which clients may not be aware, such as make-up services and the products that your salon stocks.

Adipose tissue – AD-i-pohz TISH-yoo – The layer of fat cells which lies beneath the dermis, otherwise known as the subcutaneous layer.

Adverse reaction – AD-vurss ree-AK-shuhn – When a client has a negative reaction to a hair or skin test carried out prior to any service.

Adverse skin, scalp and hair conditions – AD-vurss SKIN SKALP uhnd HAIR kuhn-DISH-uhnz – Conditions that can stop, limit or restrict a service or treatment. Examples include impetigo, scars, moles, psoriasis and alopecia.

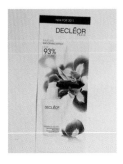

Advertising
– AD-vuh-tiyz-ing
– Forms of communication with the purpose of persuading the client to buy.

Advice – uhd-VIYSS – Knowledge given to the client after the treatment so that they can continue its benefits.

Advice on employment issues – uhd-VIYSS on im-PLOY-muhnt ISH-ooz – You can seek advice from the Citizens Advice Bureau, trade unions, a private solicitor, or a training provider (if under a government funded training scheme).

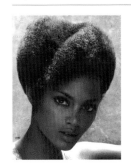

African hair type – AF-rik-uhn HAIR tiyp – This hair is usually very curly and naturally dark. African hair curl is formed because of its uneven keratinisation.

Afro look – AF-roh luuk – The natural curly look that requires shaping.

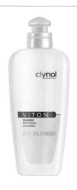

Aftercare advice – AHF-tuh-KAIR uhd-VIYSS – Advice that you should give to the client on products, maintenance of their style and further services.

Aftercare products – AHF-tuh-KAIR PROD-uhkts – Products such as dressing lotions, sprays, serums and oils that maintain a style after the client has left the salon.

AIDS – AYDZ – AIDS (acquired immune deficiency syndrome or acquired immunodeficiency syndrome) is a disease of the human immune system caused by HIV (human immunodeficiency virus).

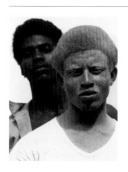

Albinism – AL-bin-izm – An inherited condition where there is the absence of pigments in the skin, hair and eyes.

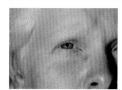

Albino hair – al-BEE-noh HAIR – Hair that contains no or very little pigment (melanin). The hair will be nearly white or a pale yellow.

Alkali – AL-kuh-liy – Alkalis have a pH value of above 7.

Alkaline perm – AL-kuh-liyn PURM – Alkaline perms have a pH of above 7 and are made up of a chemical ingredient called ammonium thioglycolate. These perms are designed to give a firm, springy curl.

Allergen – AL-uh-juhn – A substance that causes your immune system to react abnormally.

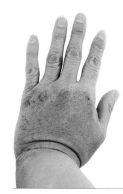

Allergic contact dermatitis – uh-LURJ-ik KON-takt dur-muh-TIYT-iss – A body reaction to an irritant, caused by exposure to sensitising agents. In many cases the sensitivity will last indefinitely.

Allergic reaction – uh-LUR-jik ree-AK-shuhn – When the client experiences a reaction to a product, you will see redness, soreness, swelling or itchiness.

A

Aloe vera shampoo – AL-oh VAIR-uh sham-POO – A mild natural base shampoo that is ideal for healthy hair and scalps; it can be used on a frequent basis.

Alopecia areata – al-uh-PEE-shuh a-REE-uh-tuh – Hair loss in patches, or baldness – whether the hair will grow back or not depends on the cause of the hair loss.

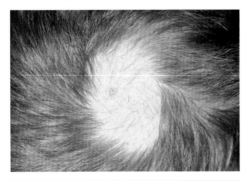

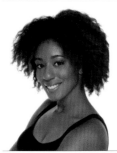

Alopecia totalis – al-uh-PEE-shuh toh-TAH-liss – Complete hair loss, sometimes including the eyebrows and eyelashes.

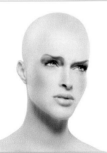

Alpha keratin – ALF-uh KE-ruh-tin – Unstretched hair in its natural state, before it has been styled.

Alum powder – AL-uhm POW-duh – Used in barbering – put it onto a small piece of damp cotton wool to stop bleeding.

Amino acid – uh-MEEN-oh ASS-id – The building block of hair.

Ammonia – uh-MOH-nee-uh – A colourless pungent gas. An alkaline ingredient used in some permanent hair colours.

Ammonium thioglycolate – uh-MOH-nee-uhm thiy-oh-GLIY-kuh-layt – The chemical most frequently used in alkaline perms to break the disulphide bonds – also used in hair depilatories.

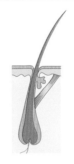

Anagen – ANN-uh-jin – The active growing stage of the hair growth cycle, which can last from 1.5 to 7 years.

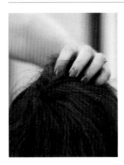

Analysis – uh-NAL-uh-siss – A full assessment of the condition of the hair and scalp by doing a visual check and manual testing to ensure there are no factors that would prevent a service from taking place.

Anaphylactic shock – AN-uh-fi-LAK-tik SHOK – An extreme allergic reaction which can be fatal.

Androgenic alopecia – an-druh-JEN-ik a-luh-PEE-shuh – Commonly known as male pattern baldness – a hereditary condition where the hair recedes at the front hairline and thins at the crown.

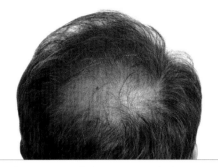

Aniline – AN-uh-liyn or AN-uh-leen – A substance used in the manufacture of hair dyes, aniline is a colourless oily liquid present in coal tar.

Anterior – an-TEER-ree-uh – Near the front.

Antibacterial – an-tee-bak-TEER-ee-uhl – A substance that prevents or stops the growth of bacteria.

Antioxidant – ann-tee-OKS-id-uhnt – A substance that stops the oxidation process after a chemical treatment.

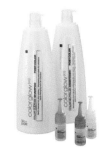

Antioxidant conditioner – ann-tee-OKS-id-uhnt kuhn-DISH-uh-nuh – A conditioner applied to the hair after a chemical service to stop the oxidation process of chemical services.

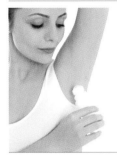

Antiperspirant – ann-tee-PURSS-puh-ruhnt – Used to reduce underarm perspiration.

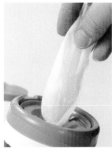

Antiseptic – an-tee-SEP-tik – A substance that will reduce the growth of micro-organisms that cause diseases.

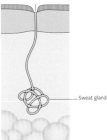

Sweat gland

Apocrine gland
– AP-uh-kreen or AP-uh-krin gland – Sweat glands composed of a coiled secretory portion located at the junction of the dermis and subcutaneous fat.

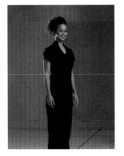

Appearance
– uh-PEER-ruhnss – How you present yourself in the salon environment.

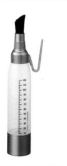

Applicator bottle – APP-li-kay-tuh BOTL – A bottle designed to apply neutraliser or a colour product with a liquid-like consistency.

Appointment – uh-POYNT-muhnt – A pre-arranged service booked for a scheduled day and time.

Appointment details – uh-POYNT-muhnt DEE-taylz – The client's name and contact details, what service they are having, the date and time, and the member of staff carrying out the service.

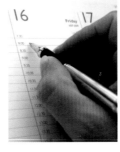

Appointment system – uh-POYNT-muhnt SISS-tuhm – A method used for recording client appointment bookings – it could be on a computer or in a book.

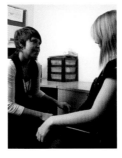

Appraisal
– uh-PRAYZ-uhl – A method by which the job performance of an employee is evaluated (generally in terms of quality, quantity, cost and time), normally conducted by the manager or supervisor.

Appropriate language – uh-PROHP-ree-uht LANG-gwij – Suitable language that helps you to communicate effectively with clients. You should not use words that are too technical. Appropriate language is always clear, polite and friendly.

Arrector pili muscle – uh-REK-tuh PILL-ee MUSS-uhl – A muscle which connects the follicle to the dermis. When this muscle is stimulated, the hairs stand up and cause goose bumps.

Arteriole – ah-TEER-ree-ohl – A tiny artery.

Artery – AH-tuh-ree – Blood vessels that carry blood away from the heart.

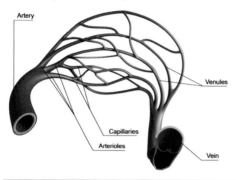

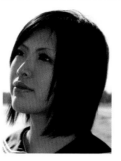

Asian hair – AY-shuhn HAIR – Also known as mongoloid; it is usually very straight.

Assembly point – uh-SEM-blee POYNT – The designated meeting point in the event of an emergency evacuation.

Assessment – uh-SESS-muhnt – An evaluation or judgement of a candidate's work performance. There are several methods of assessment, eg oral questions, written questions, witness testimonies, and assessment of prior learning and/or experience.

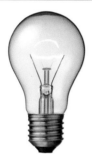

Artificial light – ah-tuh-FISH-uhl LIYT – Light that is not sunlight.

Assignment – uh-SIYN-muhnt – A set task or practical activity.

Asthma – AS-muh or AS-thmuh – A disorder of the respiratory system which causes the airways to narrow, leaving the person breathless and wheezy.

Aseptic – ay-SEP-tik – A bacteria-free area; always try to work in an area like this. This can be achieved by thorough cleaning, wearing gloves, sterilising equipement and disposing of waste properly.

Astringent – uh-STRIN-juhnt – A product that is used on the hair with a stimulating effect.

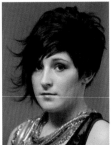

Asymmetric
– ay-sim-ET-rik –
When a style is longer on one side than the other.

Athlete's foot – ATH-leets FUUT – Athlete's foot (also known as ringworm of the foot and tinea pedis) is a fungal infection of the skin that causes scaling, flaking and itch of affected areas.

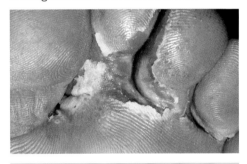

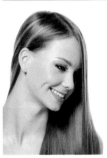

Attachment methods –
uh-TACH-muhnt METH-udz –
The different methods for hair extensions: hot fusion, cold fusion, wefts and plaiting. Hot fusion uses hot glue to attach the extensions. With cold fusion, the extensions are attached by using keratin-based polymer. Wefts are extensions that are sewn in to form small cornrows. With plaiting, extension hair is plaited together with human hair.

Attachment systems – uh-TACH-muhnt SISS-tuhmz – Methods of attaching added hair. Some examples are glue in, dip in, grip in, bonded, sewn in and plaited in.

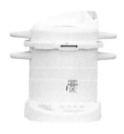

Autoclave –
OR-toh-klayv –
The most effective method of sterilisation. The water inside the autoclave is heated to 121°C, producing high temperature steam which destroys all micro-organisms.

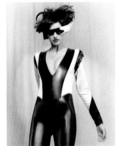

Avant-garde –
AV-o(ng)-GAHD –
A style, look or image that is ahead of the times, usually worn or produced by the leaders of fashion, before it becomes fashionable.

Azo dye – A-zoh or AY-zoh DIY – A synthetic dye, found in temporary colours, that only coats the surface of the hair.

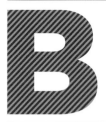

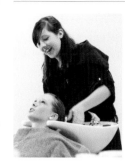

Backwash basin
– BAK-wosh BAY-suhn – Where the client sits in the chair and the head lies back into the basin; when shampooing, the client's face will not get wet using this method.

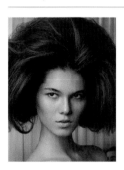

Back-brushing
– BAK-brush-ing – You will use this technique to give height and volume to hairstyles. Back-brushing is achieved by brushing the hair backwards from the points of the hair to the roots. A dressing out technique with a brush, for giving root lift and/or volume to the hair.

Backcomb taper – BAK-kohm TAY-puh – When backcombed hair is dressed into a point.

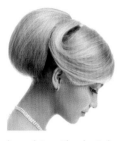

Backcombing
– BAK-kohm-ing – A dressing out technique with a comb, for giving root lift and/or volume to the hair.

Bacteria – bak-TEER-ee-uh – Micro-organisms that are responsible for infections.

Bad breath – BAD BRETH – Noticeably unpleasant odours exhaled in breathing – another term for this is halitosis.

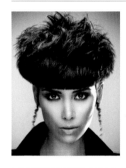

Balance – BAL-uhnss – When the hair is even on both sides.

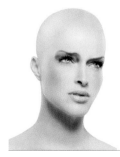

Baldness – BORLD-nuhss – Partial or complete lack of hair.

Banding – BAND-ing – Where the colour of an area of the hair is different from the rest of the hair; this usually occurs when the colour is overlapped on the previous colour.

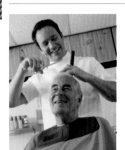

Barber – BAH-buh – A person who carries out services on male clients, for example haircuts, facial massage or shaving.

Barber's comb – BAH-buhz KOHM – A very fine and flexible comb used for cutting short hairs at the neck area.

Barber's rash – BAH-buhz RASH – Also known as sycosis barbae or barber's itch – this is the inflammation of the hair follicles caused by bacterial infection in the beard area.

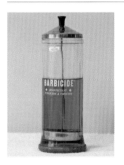

Barbicide – BAH-buh-siyd – A brand name for a disinfectant; an effective form of sterilisation is achieved when the tools are completely immersed in the chemical for the specified length of time.

Barrel curl – BA-ruhl KURL – Soft-centred, loose and springy curls that stand away from the head.

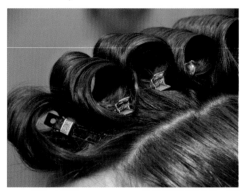

Barrier cream – BA-ree-uh KREEM – A thick protective cream on the hairline of the client, which acts as an invisible coating to protect the skin from irritation and to prevent chemicals harming the skin.

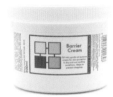

Basal layer – BAY-suhl LAY-uh – The deepest layer of the epidermis.

Base shade – BAYSS shayd – The natural colour of a client's hair; also known as depth.

Baseline – BAYSS-liyn – The perimeter line of the hairstyle.

Basic structure of the hair – BAYSS-ik STRUK-chuh uhv dhuh HAIR – The basic structure of the hair is made up of the cuticle, cortex and medulla.

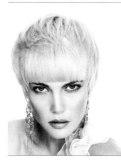

Basic uniform layer – BAYSS-ik YOON-i-form LAY-uh – All the sections of the hair are cut to the same length.

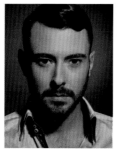

Beard – BEERD – The facial hair on a man that can be cut into a variety of shapes and can enhance the wearer's appearance.

Beard clippings – BEERD KLIP-ingz – Clippings of hair from the facial area.

Beauty therapist – BYOO-tee THERR-uh-pist – A person who is qualified to carry out a variety of treatments within a beauty salon or spa, for example facial cleansing or a body massage.

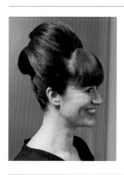

Beehive – BEE-hiyv – An updo that resembles a beehive/horizontal roll.

Behaviour – bi-HAYV-ee-uh – A person's words and actions; good manners and treating people with respect are essential.

Behavioural expectations – bi-HAYV-ee-uh-ruhl ek-spek-TAY-shuhnz – You will be expected to work co-operatively with others, and following salon requirements.

Benefit – BEN-uh-fit – The advantage of the product or service.

Benefits of effective team working – BEN-uh-fits uhv i-FEK-tive TEEM WUR-king – The benefits include: client satisfaction, personal and team achievement, positive salon reputation, repeat business, staff motivation and morale, and harmony within the working environment.

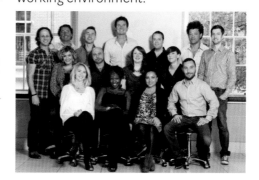

Beta keratin – BEE-tuh KE-ruh-tin – This is when the hair has been stretched, fully dried and allowed to cool into a new shape.

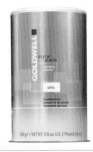

Bleach – BLEECH – A product used to lighten the hair.

Bleaching – BLEE-ching – The process of lightening the hair, by changing the melanin to colourless oxymelanin.

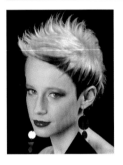

Block colour – BLOK KUH-luh – A colour applied to block sections of the hair.

Block colouring – BLOK KUH-luh-ring – Colouring areas of hair in a way that is intended to enhance the style of the cut.

Blockage – BLOK-ij – When the basin will not drain of its water due to an obstruction.

Blocked nape – BLOKT nayp – Cutting the hair straight across in a definite line where the hairline meets the back of the neck. It is sometimes also referred to as 'squaring off' the nape.

Blood capillary – BLUD kuh-PIL-uh-ree – The smallest blood vessel that is one cell thick. It allows the exchange of various substances, such as oxygen and nutrients into the cells, and carbon dioxide and waste out of the cells.

Blood vessels – BLUD VESS-uhlz – Carry blood around the body.

Blot – BLOT – The process of removing excess moisture from the hair after rinsing, using towels, cotton wool or paper towels.

Blot dry – BLOT driy – Soak up excess water using cotton wool, without rubbing the hair.

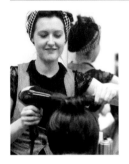

Blow dry – BLOH driy – This is achieved by using an electrical hand-held hairdryer, to create a style.

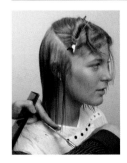

Blunt cutting – BLUNT KUT-ing – The most common cutting technique, sometimes called club cutting. The hair is combed and held with even tension before cutting; the ends of the hair are cut blunt and very heavy.

Body heat – BOD-ee HEET – Given off naturally by the client, this can affect some hair services and needs to be taken into consideration.

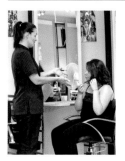

Body language – BOD-ee LANG-gwij – Consists of your posture, gestures, facial expressions and eye movements.

Body odour – BOD-ee OH-duh – Body odour, sometimes abbreviated as B.O., is the smell of bacteria growing on the body. The bacteria multiply rapidly in the presence of sweat, but sweat itself is almost completely odourless to humans.

Bonding – BOND-ing – A method of applying wefts or hair extensions using a glue or an adhesive to secure them to the existing hair.

Bone structure of the face – BOHN STRUK-chuh uhv dhuh FAYSS – The bones of the face include the mandible, maxillae, zygomatic and frontal.

Bones of the head and neck – BOHNZ uhv dhuh HED uhnd NEK – The main bones in the head are the occipital, frontal, parietal, temporal, sphenoid, and ethmoid bones; the bones in the neck are the cervical vertebrae.

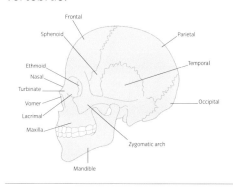

Booster – BOOST-uh – A product that provides additional oxygen to speed up a chemical service.

Bouffant – BOO-fo(ng) – A hairstyle that is very full with lots of volume.

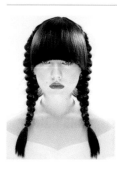

Braid – BRAYD – A method of weaving strands of hair together.

Breach of security – BREECH uhv suh-KYOO-uh-ri-tee – When someone gets in somewhere they shouldn't have been able to, for example if the salon is broken into at night.

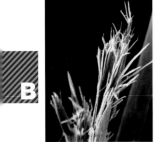

Breakage – BRAY-kij – Hair that has been damaged by excess chemical or physical treatments.

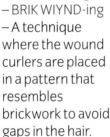

Brick winding – BRIK WIYND-ing – A technique where the wound curlers are placed in a pattern that resembles brickwork to avoid gaps in the hair. This technique is suitable for clients with fine, shorter hair.

Bristle brush – BRISSL BRUSH – Used to lather up shaving products and apply them to the face. A brush with soft bristles.

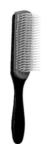

Brushes – BRUSH-iz – Include bristle, Denman, paddle, round, shaving and vented.

Budget – BUJ-it – A given amount of money within which you need to work.

Build-up – BILD-uhp – An excess of a product, built up on the hair over a period of time.

Business – BIZ-niss – An organisation engaged in the sale of goods and or services.

Business promotion – BIZ-niss pruh-MOH-shuhn – Advertising your business in a cost-effective and easy way to increase income by generating more clients.

Butterfly clamps – BUT-uh-fliy KLAMPS – A style of sectioning clips, used to hold large sections of hair apart.

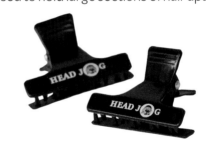

Buying signal – BIY-ing SIG-nuhl – A comment from a client, which indicates that they are thinking about buying your product or service. The most common buying signal is the question: 'How much is it?'. Others are questions or comments such as: 'What sizes does it come in?'.

By-laws – BIY-lohz – Local laws passed from a higher authority and can vary from place to place. Contact your local HSE for more information about your area's by-laws.

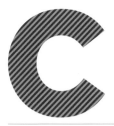

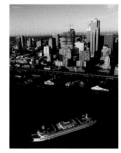

Career opportunities – kuh-REER op-uh-TYOON-it-eez – The roles and places in which you may work once you are qualified.

Calcium hydroxide-based relaxer (non-lye) – KALSS-ee-uhm hyd-ROKS-iyd-BAYST ri-LAKS-uh -- non-LIY – A chemical used in a relaxer, which causes less irritation for the client; it is ideal for clients who have sensitive scalps and who are sensitive to sodium hydroxide.

Calculate – KALK-yoo-layt – This is when you do some maths, eg adding up the client's bill for all the services, or when you need to work out mixing ratios.

Camomile shampoo – KAM-uh-miyl sham-POO – Made from a plant of the daisy family, this shampoo is best used on greasy hair and can brighten blonde hair.

Canities – kuh-NISH-ee-eez – The greyness or whiteness of hair with little or no pigment.

Cap weave – KAP weev – Also known as stocking cap weave – this is a wig that can be attached to existing hair.

Capillary – kuh-PIL-uh-ree – An extremely small blood vessel located within the tissues of the body; it transports blood from arteries to veins.

Cash – KASH – Banknotes and coins.

Cash equivalent – KASH i-KWIV-uh-luhnt – When a client pays with a voucher or a points system.

Cash flow forecast – KASH FLOH FOR-kahst – An estimate of when and how much money will be received and paid out of a business.

Cashing up – KASH-ing uhp – At the end of a day's business, the till is counted to see if the takings are accurate for the day.

Cashpoint – KASH poynt – Where you insert your debit/credit card and enter your PIN to obtain cash.

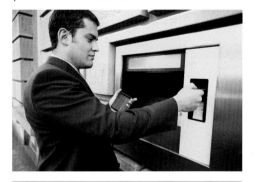

Castle serrations – KAH-suhl suh-RAY-shuhnz – Serrated scissors used for thinning or reducing the thickness of the hair.

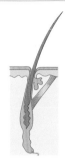

Catagen – KAT-uh-jen – In the hair growth cycle, this is the stage when the hair follicles undergo a period of change and growing stops, usually for around two weeks. This is also known as the transitional phase.

Catwalk show – KAT-work SHOH (N.B. '-walk' rhymes with 'fork') – Usually performed on a runway, it features models who are showcasing a designer's clothes or new collections.

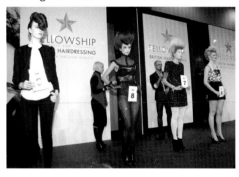

Caucasian hair – kor-KAY-zhuhn HAIR – One of the three ethnic hair types (Asian and African type are the other two). Caucasian hair is usually straight or slightly wavy and is sometimes referred to as European hair.

Caustic – KOR-stik – A chemical that will burn and cause harm to the skin.

Certificate of registration – suh-TIF-ik-uht uhv rej-iss-TRAY-shuhn – This is awarded when salon premises have been successfully inspected to ensure that they are complying with local by-laws in relation to cosmetic piercing.

Cetrimide – SET-rih-miyd – A substance used in hairspray. This chemical will help condition the hair and reduce static electricity.

Channel setting – CHAN-uhl SET-ing – A uniformed setting technique where the rollers are placed in rows or channels.

Chemical service – KEM-ikl SUR-viss – Hair services such as perming, relaxing and colouring that affect the hair structure.

Chemically treated hair – KEM-ik-lee TREET-id HAIR – Hair that has been permed, relaxed, coloured, bleached or had any other chemical treatment.

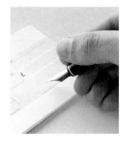

Cheque – CHEK – A form of payment for a service; cheques must be accompanied by a cheque guarantee card.

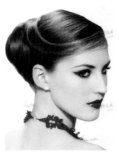

Chignon – SHEEN-YO(ng) – An elegant, sophisticated up style, where the hair is twisted into a roll or knot, usually worn between the crown and the nape area – it can be any size.

Chin curtain – CHIN KUR-tuhn – A beard shaped by facial hair growth along the lower portion of the face at the chin, following the jaw line. This can be a broad line giving a more traditional finish, or modernised with a narrow line along the jaw line.

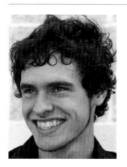

Chinstrap – CHIN-strap – A beard resembling the chinstrap of a helmet.

Chlorinated water – KLOR-in-ay-tid WOR-tuh – Water treated with chlorine, which is effective in preventing the spread of waterborne disease.

Chronic dermatitis – KRON-ik dur-muh-TIY-tiss – Caused by overexposure to an irritant over a period of time, be it days, weeks, months or years.

Cicatricial alopecia – sik-uh-TRISH-uhl al-uh-PEE-shuh – An area of baldness as a result of scarring or scar tissue.

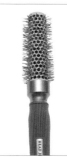

Circular brushes – SUR-kyuh-luh BRUSH-iz – Round brushes that are useful for creating curl; the smaller the brush the tighter the curl.

Circulation – surk-yuh-LAY-shuhn – The movement of substances around the body – oxygen and nutrient are transported to the cells and carbon dioxide and waste are transported from the cells.

City & Guilds – SIT-ee uhnd GILDZ – The leading awarding body in hairdressing and beauty therapy qualifications. City & Guilds offers qualifications over a range of industry sectors through colleges and training providers in many countries worldwide.

Clarifying shampoo – KLA-rif-iy-ing sham-POO – A deep-cleansing shampoo, used before applying extensions or chemical services to remove products, oils and residues from the hair.

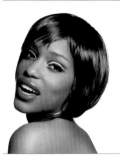

Classic look
– KLASS-ik LUUK
– A style that never dates or goes out of fashion, such as a classic bob.

Clear layer – KLEER LAY-uh – Also known as stratum lucidum, this layer of the skin sits just below the horny layer. This layer is transparent and colourless, allowing colour from below to be seen.

Client – KLIY-uhnt – A person, sometimes referred to as customer, who visits the salon for treatments. It might also be a person who is commissioning a photo shoot. They may not always be present on the day, so you need to make sure you've designed exactly what they asked for.

Client care – KLIY-uhnt KAIR – This is being able to treat the client with respect and professionalism at all times. Realising this is the key to your success.

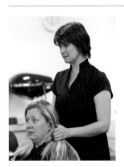

Client comfort
– KLIY-uhnt KUMF-uht – Making sure that the position of the client's head is not uncomfortable and that they are seated correctly in the chair.

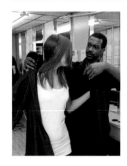

Client preparation
– KLIY-uhnt prep-uh-RAY-shuhn – Preparing the client for the service by using a gown and towels to protect the client's clothes, brushing their hair and positioning them comfortably at the basin.

Client records – KLIY-uhnt REK-ordz – A record of the client's personal details, including contact details and all services carried out.

Client rights – KLIY-uhnt RIYTS – Clients have legal rights to be protected. For example, under the Sale of Goods Act, The Supply of Goods and Services Act, it's important to know what client's rights are, and to comply with them.

Client satisfaction – KLIY-uhnt sat-is-FAK-shuhn – When the client's expectations for the service have been met by the stylist.

Client specification or brief – KLIY-uhnt spess-if-i-KAY-shuhn or BREEF – A description of what the client is looking for, usually in written form.

Client's features – KLIY-uhnts FEE-chuhz – Eyes, ears, cheekbones and other factors that are taken into consideration when producing styles for the client.

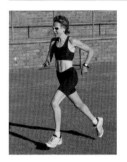

Client's lifestyle – KLIY-uhnts LIYF-styl – Factors in the client's life that influence the choice of hairstyle; eg, a client who works in the fashion industry may wish to match their image with the latest fashions.

Client's requirements – KLIY-uhnts ruh-KWIY-uh-muhnts – Any requests from the client; it may not always be possible to meet their needs, so a compromise may be needed.

Climazone – KLIY-muh-zohn – An electrical piece of equipment that is used to speed up chemical services.

Clinical waste – KLIN-ikl WAYST – Waste that has been soiled with bodily fluids or skin tissue.

Clip-on extensions – KLIP-on iks-TEN-shuhnz – Temporary hair extensions with clips or combs attached; the wefts are normally pre-coloured.

Clipper over comb – KLIP-uh OH-vuh KOHM – A method of cutting the hair: the hair is combed in an upward direction and protrudes through the comb; the hair is then cut with the clipper blades.

Clippers – KLIP-uhz – Electrical equipment with graded attachments, used when barbering.

Clockspring curl – KLOK-spring KURL – A pin curl that is wound into a coil forming a clockspring curl; the curl sits flat on the head, is tight and closely coiled at the ends of the hair, and gradually gets looser the root area.

Closed questions – KLOHZD KWES-chuhnz – Questions that lead to yes and no answers, for example 'Would you like styling spray on your hair?'.

Closing the sale – KLOH-zing dhuh SAYL – Gaining agreement from the client to buy.

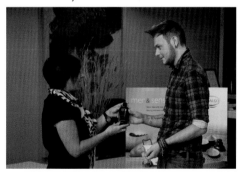

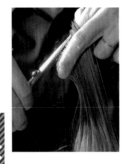

Club cutting or blunt cutting
– KLUB KUT-ing or BLUNT KUT-ing – The most basic way of cutting sections of hair is straight across, parallel to the index and middle fingers.

Co-operation – koh-op-uh-RAY-shuhn – Working together with others to achieve common goals.

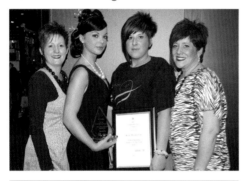

Coarse hair – KORSS HAIR – Thick, strong hair, with a large diameter.

Coconut shampoo – KOH-kuh-nut sham-POO – A shampoo that is best used on dry hair; it contains an emollient which helps to regain its elasticity.

Code of practice – KOHD uhv PRAK-tiss – Set rules of working, laid out by the industry or by the workplace itself.

Cohesive setting – koh-HEE-siv SET-ing – A setting technique for either directional or brick setting.

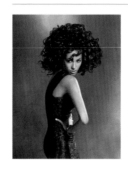

Coiffure – kwa-FYOO-uh – The finished hairstyle that has been arranged and is attractive.

Cold attachment methods for hair extensions – KOHLD uh-TACH-muhnt METH-uhdz fuh HAIR iks-TEN-shuhnz – There are several methods for attaching hair extensions; these include cold fusion, sewing, fusing, self-adhesive, clip-in and plaiting.

Cold fusion extension systems – KOHLD FYOO-zhuhn iks-TEN-shuhn SISS-tuhmz – A system of attaching extensions by using adhesives, adhesive strips and tapes; it can be used on any hair type.

Cold permanent waving lotion – KOHLD PUR-muh-nuhnt WAKS-ing LOH-shuhn – A type of perm lotion that does not depend on heat for its activation.

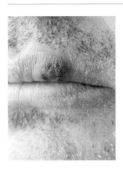

Cold sore –
KOHLD SOR
– Small, blister-like wounds that usually appear around the mouth. They are caused by the herpes simplex virus.

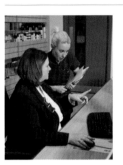

Colleagues
– KOL-eegz –
Someone you work with.

Colour bands – KUH-luh BANDZ – Dark or intense lines/patches of colour, often resulting from overlapping colour.

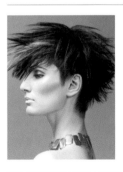

Colour correction
– KUH-luh kuh-REK-shuhn
– Changing coloured hair that has already been coloured.

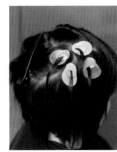

Colour cups
– KUH-luh KUPS
– A technique for creating a number of multi-coloured highlighting effects.

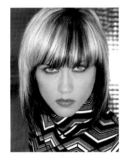

Colour depth
– KUH-luh DEPTH
– Lightness or darkness of the hair, eg 2–9 on the international colour chart system.

Colour development strand test – KUH-luh duh-VEL-uhp-muhnt STRAND TEST – Also known as a strand test, this is carried out during the processing stage to check the development of the colour or lightener.

Colour fade – KUH-luh FAYD – When hair colour gradually appears weaker.

Colour filling – KUH-luh FIL-ing – The process of pre-pigmenting the hair and then adding the required depth.

Colour mapping

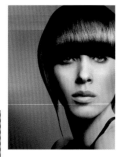

Colour mapping – KUH-luh MAP-ing – Accentuating a haircut by placing colours in the hair to highlight an area of the cut, for example blonde on top with a darker bottom section will add density to the hair, as a darker colour at the nape area will give the impression of adding density to the hair.

Colour pigment – KUH-luh PIG-muhnt – There are two colour pigments that give the hair and skin their colour: pheomelanin (red and yellow) and eumelanin (black and brown).

Colour remover – KUH-luh ri-MOO-vuh – A product that removes artificial colour and/or tone.

Colour spectrum – KUH-luh SPEK-truhm – A range of colours that makes up white sunlight: red, orange, yellow, green, blue, indigo and violet.

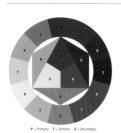

P = Primary   T = Tertiary   S = Secondary

Colour star/wheel – KUH-luh STAH/WEEL – A circle of colour that is divided into six equal portions: three from the primary colours and three from the secondary colours.

Colour test – KUH-luh TEST – A test on a small cutting of the hair to determine if a colour is suitable and achievable.

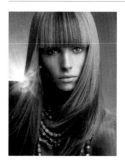

Colour tone – KUH-luh TOHN – The colours you see in the hair, for example red, copper, golden.

Colourant – KUH-luh-ruhnt – A type of colour substance used on the hair.

Colouring materials – KUH-luh-ring muh-TEER-ee-uhlz – Materials used to colour the hair, such as packets, foils, wraps, meche and cotton wool.

Colouring products – KUH-luh-ring PROD-uhkts – Products used to colour the hair, such as colours, bleach, high-lift tint and hydrogen peroxide.

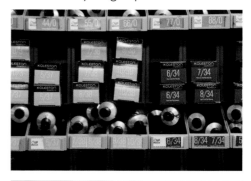

Comb twist – KOHM TWIST – A flat twist that sits along the scalp and is created with a comb.

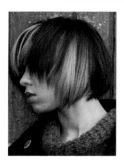

Combination – kom-bi-NAY-shuhn – When more than one technique is used on the same client.

Combustible – kuhm-BUST-uhbl – The tendency of something to react with oxygen and catch fire.

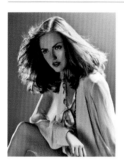

Commercial – kuh-MUR-shuhl – An image that clients would want to wear on a regular basis.

Commercial look – kuh-MUR-shuhl LUUK – An everyday look that is suitable for many different people and is easy to wear.

Commercial viability – kuh-MUR-shuhl viy-uh-BIL-it-ee – Making sure you don't spend too much time on tasks. If you take too long doing one thing, your salon loses money because you could be doing something else more valuable for the business. Remember that time is money and you're being paid to be efficient.

Commission – kuh-MISH-uhn – An incentive from your employer to encourage you to make recommendations and boost your monthly wage, as well as the salon's profits.

Commission basis – kuh-MISH-uhn BAY-siss – When stylists receive a percentage of the sale value that they create.

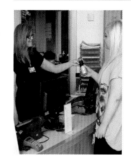

Communication – kuh-myoo-ni-KAY-shuhn – Giving or exchanging of information, signals or messages through speech, gestures or writing.

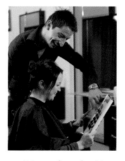

Communication skills – kuh-myoo-ni-KAY-shuhn SKILZ – The ability to pass on information accurately by listening carefully, and talking and writing clearly. You should be polite, friendly, helpful and respectful when communicating with clients.

Compensation – kom-pen-SAY-shuhn – A form of insurance that provides wage replacement and medical benefits to employees who have incurred work-related injuries.

Competition work – kom-puh-TISH-uhn WURK – Competing against each other to achieve a common goal.

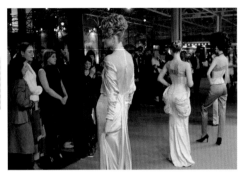

Complaint – kuhm-PLAYNT – When a client is not happy with a service; you need to remain calm and courteous at all times.

Complementary colours – kom-pluh-MEN-tree KUH-luhz – Colours that go together well.

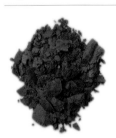

Compound colour – KOM-pownd KUH-luh – A mixture of vegetable and mineral dyes.

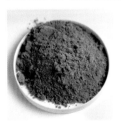

Compound henna – KOM-pownd HEN-uh – This product is not compatible with modern hairdressing chemical products; compound henna contains a combination of vegetable henna and metallic salts.

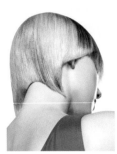

Concave baseline – KONG-KAYV BAYSS-liyn – When the baseline is cut to curve inwards or downwards towards the sides, such as on a bob, where the baseline curves down towards the sides.

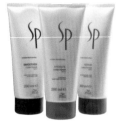

Conditioner – kuhn-DISH-uhn-uh – A product that helps the hair to look shiny and feel silky, and smooths down the cuticle.

Conditioning massage movements – kuhn-DISH-uhn-ing MASS-ahzh MOOV-muhnts – Effleurage and petrissage are massage movements that are used when conditioning the hair.

Conditioning products – kuhn-DISH-uhn-ing PROD-uhkts – Surface conditioner, penetrating conditioner and scalp treatments – each has a different purpose.

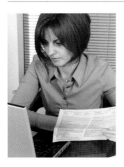

Confidential information – kon-fi-DEN-shuhl in-fuh-MAY-shuhn – Private information that must not be passed on.

Confidentiality – kon-fi-den-shee-AL-it-ee – All employers have a duty to their staff and customers to maintain confidentiality relating to their personal details. All employees are responsible for adhering to and maintaining the salon's confidentiality. Confidentiality is a legal requirement under the Data Protection Act.

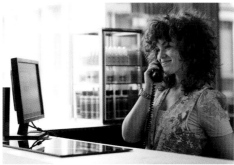

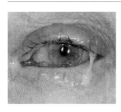

Conjunctivitis – kuhn-junk-ti-VIY-tiss – Inflammation and infection of the eyes.

Consultation – kon-sul-TAY-shuhn – A discussion between the stylist and a client to determine the services and treatments that reflect the client's requirements.

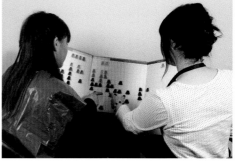

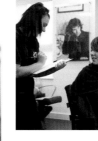

Consultation techniques – kon-sul-TAY-shuhn tek-NEEKS – Methods of finding out relevant information from your client so you can plan and perform a service.

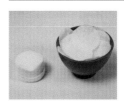

Consumables – kuhn-SYOOM-uhblz – An item which cannot be reused, eg a cotton bud.

Consumer – kuhn-SYOO-muh – The client buying the treatment, service or product.

Consumer and retail legislation –
kuhn-SYOO-muh uhnd REE-tayl lej-iss-LAY-shuhn – The different Acts in place are to protect the client, for example the Trades Descriptions Act, the Prices Act, the Sale and Supply of Goods Act, the Consumer Protection Act, the Consumer Safety Act, and the Data Protection Act.

Consumer Protection Act – kuhn-SYOO-muh pruh-TEK-shuhn akt – A law that protects clients from unsafe products and misleading prices.

Contact dermatitis – KON-takt
durm-uh-TIY-tiss – You can avoid this condition by making sure that you always use disposable non-latex gloves. Some of the symptoms are dryness, redness and itching, and this can develop into flaking, cracking, bleeding, swelling and blistering of the hands. Always rinse and dry your hands thoroughly after washing, and moisturise them.

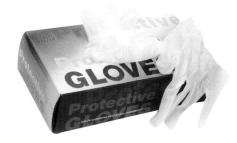

Contagious – kuhn-TAY-juhss –
A disease, such as impetigo, that can be spread from one person to another, through either direct or indirect contact.

Contaminated waste – kuhn-TAM-in-ay-tid WAYST – Consumables that have been soiled with bodily fluids; this type of waste requires special disposal methods.

Contamination – kuhn-ta-mi-NAY-shuhn – The presence of something unwanted that might be harmful.

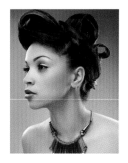

Contemporary look – kuhn-TEM-puh-ruh-ree LUUK – Modern day hair-up styles; these will include the use of knots, twists, plaits and weaving.

Contingency plan – kuhn-TIN-juhn-see PLAN – Back-up or secondary plan.

Continuing professional development (CPD) – kuhn-TIN-yoo-uhl pruh-FESH-uh-nuhl duh-VEL-uhp-muhnt – Keeping your skills and knowledge in your chosen profession up to date, by attending courses, workshops, lectures, etc.

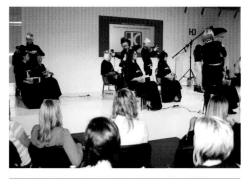

Contra-action – KON-truh-AK-shuhn – An unwanted reaction occurring during or after treatment.

Contra-indication – KON-truh in-di-KAY-shuhn – A disease, hair disorder, infection of the scalp, infection of the skin, breakage of the hair or infestation, which prevents a service or treatment from taking place.

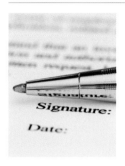

Contract of employment – KON-trakt uhv im-PLOY-muhnt – An agreement between an employer and an employee, setting out the terms and conditions of the job.

Contractor – kuhn-TRAK-tuh – A person who isn't directly employed by a business but does have a contract with them to complete work by a set deadline. For example, a builder.

Contractual agreement – kuhn-TRAK-tyoo-uhl uh-GREE-muhnt – This is a verbal or written agreement undertaken by you, the salon and the client to carry out the agreed standard of service, providing the benefits discussed at the agreed price.

Contrast – KON-trahst – A noticeable difference between colours, eg black and white.

Control – kuhn-TROHL – The elimination or reduction of the risk to acceptable levels.

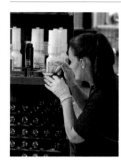

Control of Substances Hazardous to Health (COSHH) – kuhn-TROHL uhv SUB-stuhn-siz HAZ-uh-duhss tuh HELTH -- KOSH – This is the legislation that requires employers to assess the risks from harmful products and take safety measures. Store in a locked cupboard, handle according to the manufacturer's instructions, use in a ventilated area and dispose of chemicals according to the manufacturer's instructions and local by-laws.

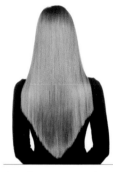

Convex baseline – KON-VEKS BAYSS-liyn – When the hair is cut longer at the middle back section and shorter at the sides.

Cool tones – KOOL TOHNZ – Tones such as green, violet and blue.

Copyright – KO-pee-riyt – The legal right that gives the creator of a piece of work control over how it is used by others.

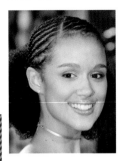

Cornrows – KORN-rohz – Also known as canerows. These are three stranded plaits that sit on their own base and form small tracks of raised scalp plaits that can be sectioned to go in any direction required. They can be used to form tracks to sew wefts of hair onto them.

Correct posture – kuh-REKT POSS-chuh – Positioning yourself correctly to prevent fatigue and long-term injury.

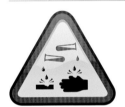

Corrosive – kuh-ROH-siv – A corrosive substance will destroy or damage what it comes into contact with. The main hazards to people include damage to the eyes, the skin and the tissue under the skin.

Cortex – KOR-teks – The main layer in the structure of the hair, which lies under the cuticle (the disulphide bonds are found here) and colour pigments.

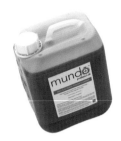

COSHH – KOSH – The Control of Substances Hazardous to Health Regulations. See www.hse.gov.uk for more information.

Cosmetic Products Regulations 2008 – KOZ-me-tik PROD-uhkts reg-yuh-LAY-shuhnz TOO-OH-OH-AYT – All cosmetic products supplied in the UK, whether for consumer or professional use, must comply with the Cosmetic Products (Safety) Regulations 2008. The regulations require that finished cosmetic products must undergo a safety assessment by a suitably qualified person before they can be placed on the market.

Cost-effective – KOST-if-FEKT-iv – Achieving a style at good value for money.

Courteous – KURT-ee-uhss – Having good manners and being polite.

Courteous behaviour – KURT-ee-uhss bi-HAY-vee-uh – This means treating your client politely and showing them respect.

Cowlick – KOW-lik – A hair growth pattern normally found at the front of the forehead.

Creating curl – kree-AY-ting KURL – The size of the brush or roller will determine how much curl is produced. The smaller the brush or roller, the curlier the finish.

Creating movement – kree-AY-ting MOOV-muhnt – Determined by the direction of the style and the amount of waves and curls the style has.

Creating volume – kree-AY-ting VOL-yoom – Created by the direction at which the hair is held at the roots when drying. The finished result will be bouncy at the roots.

Creative skills – kree-AY-tiv SKILZ – Using your imagination and artistic flair when creating new fashion trends.

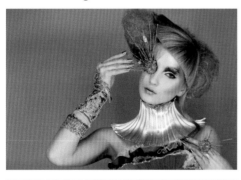

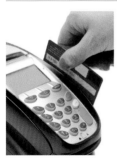

Credit card – KRED-it KAHD – A means of making payment without using cash.

Creeping oxidation – KREE-ping oks-id-AY-shuhn – Occurs when residues of chemicals are left in the hair. The chemical reactions they produce carry on working and will cause damage to the hair.

Crepe hair – KRAYP or KREP HAIR – A man-made fibre placed on the ends of the hair and used as a winding aid in perm winding.

Crew cut – KROO KUT – A hairstyle for men that is short and spiky.

Crimping irons – KRIM-ping IY-uhnz (N.B. 'irons' rhymes with 'lions') – Heated styling equipment with corrugated plates used to create zig zag patterns in the hair.

Croquignole winding – KROH-kuh-nohl WIYN-ding – A method of winding the hair from points to roots. This method is used when volume, lift and movement are required.

Cross-check – KROSS-CHEK – If the hair is cut using vertical sections, you would use horizontal sections to cross-check the hair.

Cross-contamination – KROSS-kuhn-ta-mi-NAY-shuhn – When micro-organisms are allowed to come into contact with a surface/substance.

Cross-infection – KROSS-in-FEK-shuhn – When the carrier of a disease passes it to someone else.

Cross-infestation – KROSS in-fes-TAY-shuhn – When an infestation of parasites, such as head lice, is passed from one person to another.

Crown – KROWN – The area at the top of the head.

Cultural and fashion trends – KUHL-chuh-ruhl uhnd FASH-uhn TRENDZ – Looks that either complement fashion changes or support cultural occasions or needs.

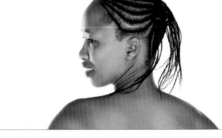

Curl base – KURL BAYSS – A section of hair where the curl sits on its own base.

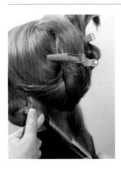

Curling tong – KUR-ling TONG – A heated styling tool used to temporarily curl the hair.

Curly hair – KUR-lee HAIR – Hair that has a natural, uneven distribution of keratin along the hair shaft.

Customer – KUSS-tuh-muh – A person who isn't necessarily a client but has come into the salon to enquire about the services offered or to buy a product.

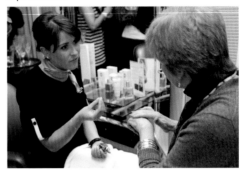

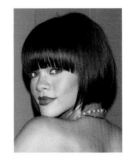

Current look – KUH-ruhnt LUUK – A commercial style that is currently fashionable. It might be a style that a celebrity has, so clients may request.

Curtain rail – KUR-tuhn RAYL – A narrow beard following the mandible.

Custom blended hair – KUSS-tuhm BLEN-did HAIR – Added hair is blended to match the client's hair colour.

Cuticle – KYOO-tikl – The outer layer of the hair, made up of overlapping scales of keratin.

Cuticle scales – KYOO-tikl SKAYLZ – The outer layer of the hair shaft, overlapping like the tiles on a roof to protect the internal part of the hair structure.

Cutting terminology – KUT-ing turm-in-OL-uh-jee – Different types of cutting techniques, eg one length, long graduation, short graduation and uniform layers.

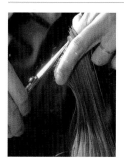

Cutting angle – KUT-ing ANG-guhl – The angle at which the hair is held and cut.

Cylindrical-shaped objects – sil-IN-drikl-SHAYPT OB-jikts – Objects that can be used for creative setting, eg chopsticks, bendies, velcro rollers, spiral rods, straws, etc.

Cutting collar – KUT-ing KO-luh – Used to protect the client from hair clippings.

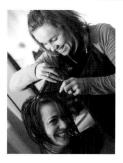

Cutting method – KUT-ing METH-uhd – A sequence of cutting techniques.

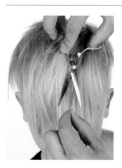

Cutting technique – KUT-ing tek-NEEK – A special cutting skill for producing a specific result.

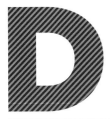

Damaged hair – DAM-ijd HAIR – This condition is where the hair is torn or split and can be identified by rough raised cuticles, loss of moisture and dry and porous hair. Normally, the cause would be harsh physical damage or chemical treatments.

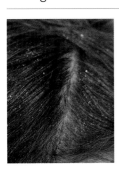

Dandruff – DAN-druhf – Skin cells on the hair, which look like small white flakes.

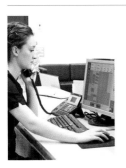

Data Protection Act – DAY-tuh pruh-TEK-shuhn akt – The law that controls the way in which information is stored. For example, clients have the right to see the information that you have on your system about them and to correct anything that they feel is inaccurate.

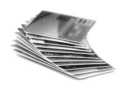

Debit card – DEB-it KAHD – A means of making payment without cash; the money instantly leaves the client's bank account.

Debris – DEB-ree – This is the excess of a material that is not used, eg excess glue when applying hair extensions.

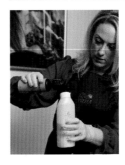

Decant – dee-KANT – To pour liquid from one container to another, usually from a larger container to a smaller container.

Decolouring/colour reduction – dee-KUH-luh-ring/KUH-luh ri-DUK-shuhn – Removing artificial/synthetic colour from the hair.

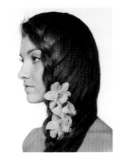

Decoration – dek-uh-RAY-shuhn – Ornamentation that is used to enhance the finished look, such as flowers or jewels.

Defects – DEE-fekts – In products, this applies to the product and packaging, such as leaking containers or loose packaging.

Demonstration – dem-uhn-STRAY-shuhn – A physical display that may include explanation or description.

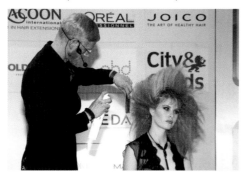

Denman brush – DEN-muhn BRUSH – A flat brush that is used to produce straight smooth styles.

Density – DEN-sit-ee – The amount of follicles in a given area of the skin, which will affect the amount of hair – sparse hair has low density, whereas abundant hair has high density.

Deodorant – dee-OH-duh-ruhnt – Used to prevent underarm and foot odour.

Depilatory – duh-PIL-uh-tree – Hair removal.

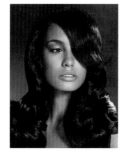

Depth – DEPTH – The lightness or darkness of the client's hair colour.

Dermal papilla – DUR-muhl puh-PIL-uh – The dermal papilla fits into the hair bulb and contains the blood and nerve supply, which nourish the cells around the hair bulb for growth.

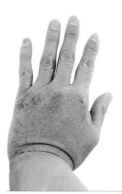

Dermatitis – dur-muh-TIY-tiss – A common skin condition suffered by hairdressers, when wet work and contact with chemicals cause soreness, redness and itchiness to the skin.

Dermatologist – dur-muh-TOL-uh-jist – A specialist who diagnoses and treats skin disorders.

Dermis – DUR-miss – The layer under the epidermis, which contains collagen and elastin fibres.

Design objective – di-ZIYN uhb-JEK-tiv – The aim or desired end result for the image.

Design plans – di-ZIYN PLANZ – A detailed outline of the selected image, including accessories, clothes, any other media, timescale for delivery, etc.

Design principles – di-ZIYN PRIN-sip-uhlz – The image's balance, weight, angles, media and colour, etc.

Detergents – di-TUR-juhnts – Used in shampoos as a wetting agent to help reduce the surface tension of the hair, allowing the water to penetrate the hair more easily when shampooing.

Developer – duh-VEL-uh-puh – A product, such as hydrogen peroxide, added to colours and bleach to make the cuticles swell.

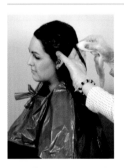

Development strand test – duh-VEL-uhp-muhnt STRAND TEST – A test carried out on the hair during the colouring process to check whether the desired development of colour has been achieved.

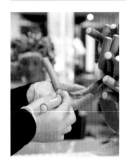

Development test curl – duh-VEL-uhp-muhnt TEST KURL – A test that is carried out on the hair during the perming process to check whether the desired development of the curl has been reached.

Development time – duh-VEL-uhp-muhnt TIYM – The time given by the manufacturers for a colour or perm to develop.

Dexterity – deks-TERR-it-ee – Precise and flexible handling.

Diagnosis – diy-uhg-NOH-siss – Observing and identifying a disease or disorder.

Diamond mesh – DIY-uh-muhnd MESH – Also known as a honeycomb mesh. An arrangement of wefts (including a fine wire) appears in a diamond-shaped pattern.

Diffuse alopecia – dif-FYOOSS al-uh-PEE-shuh – Normally found in women whose hormone levels change, it involves a gradual loss/thinning of the hair.

Diffuse pigment – dif-YOOSS PIG-muhnt – The red or yellow pigment in the hair, also known as pheomelanin.

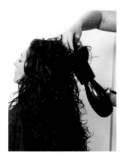

Diffuser – dif-FYOO-zuh – A plastic attachment with prongs that fits on to the hairdryer. It distributes heat so that natural hair movement and curl are encouraged as the hair is dried.

Dilated capillaries – diy-LAY-tid kuh-PILL-uh-riz – Fine red lines that show through the skin; often found on sensitive fine skin on the cheeks or around the nostrils. Sometimes referred to as thread veins.

Direction of growth – diy-REK-shuhn uhv GROHTH – The direction the hair grows up through the follicle and out on to the skin's surface.

Directional winding – duh-REK-shuhn-uhl WIYN-ding – A technique where the hair is wound in the direction in which it's going to be worn. Hair can be wound in any direction. This technique is suitable for clients with shorter hair.

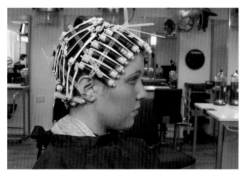

Disability discrimination – dis-uh-BIL-uh-tee dis-krim-i-NAY-shuhn – It is unlawful to discriminate against any person with a disability. For more information, see www.disability.gov.uk.

Disability Discrimination Act – dis-uh-BIL-uh-tee dis-krim-i-NAY-shuhn akt – This protects people and makes it unlawful to discriminate against a person with a disability on the grounds of his or her disability. This is in relation to recruitment, promotion, training, benefits, or terms and conditions of employment and dismissal.

Disciplinary procedure – diss-ip-LIN-uh-ree pruh-SEED-yuh – Employers use disciplinary procedures to tell employees that their performance or conduct isn't up to the expected standard, and to encourage the employee to improve.

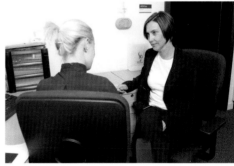

Discolouration – dis-kuh-luh-RAY-shuhn – An unwanted colour produced by a chemical – it may occur when perming over a colour.

Disconnected cut

Disconnected cut – dis-kuh-NEK-tid KUT – When one or more sections of the haircut do not connect, link or blend with adjacent sections.

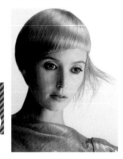

Disconnecting – dis-kuh-NEK-ting – A technique for creating long and short lengths that do not blend together.

Discrepancies – diss-KREP-uhn-sizz – A term used when handling money. The discrepancy might be an invalid credit card, invalid currency, suspected fraudulent payments using a card, etc.

Discussion – diss-KUSH-uhn – A conversation between the client and the stylist to determine the client's needs.

Disease – diz-EEZ – An abnormal condition affecting the body.

Disentangling – diss-in-TANG-gling – Combing the hair with a large tooth comb, starting at the ends of the hair and working towards the root; this method is used so that you do not damage the hair.

Disinfect – diss-in-FEKT – To destroy harmful and most other micro-organisms.

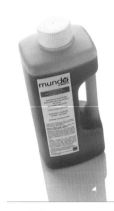

Disinfectant – diss-in-FEK-tuhnt – A chemical solution used to inhibit/kill the growth of bacteria when cleaning and sterilising tools and equipment in the salon.

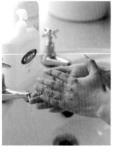

Disinfecting hands – diss-in-FEK-ting HANDZ – Washing the hands to an antiseptic level to limit the presence of bacteria.

Disinfection – diss-in-FEK-shuhn – This limits the growth of disease causing micro-organisms using chemical agents.

Display – diss-PLAY – An arrangement of products and other media to attract attention.

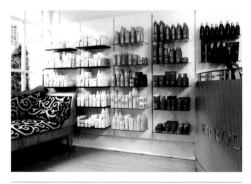

Disposables – diss-POH-zuh-buhlz – Single-use products and equipment, such as paper towels, cotton pads, orange sticks, unwashable files and buffers.

Disposal of contaminated waste – diss-POH-zuhl uhv kuhn-TAM-in-ay-tid WAYST – It will be necessary to check the correct disposal of the crystals with your local council, as occasional 'pin prick' bleeding may occur.

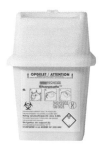

Disposal of sharps – diss-POH-zuhl uhv SHAHPS – Sharp items such as razor blades must be disposed of in a sharps box. Special arrangements are made with the local authority for incineration.

Disposal of waste – diss-POH-zuhl uhv WAYST – Everyday waste such as hair clippings, neck wool and plastic aprons should be disposed of in a lidded bin with a plastic bin liner inside it.

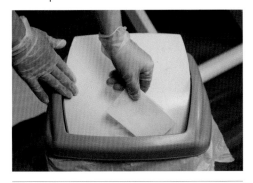

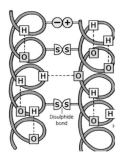

Disulphide bonds – diy-SUL-fiyd bondz – To change the hair permanently from straight to curly or curly to straight, you must change the structure of the hair. This is done by 'breaking' the disulphide bonds found in the cortex layer of the hair. Only 25–30% of these bonds should be broken during the perming process.

Diversity – diy-VUR-sit-ee – Mixture or range.

Divulge – diy-VULJ – Make known to others.

Double base – DUBL BAYSS – A colour where the base is more intensive, mainly to cover resistant white hair, eg 99/0.

Double booking – DUBL BUUK-ing – When two clients have been booked in at the same time, owing to an error in the booking system.

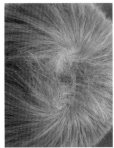

Double crown – DUBL KROWN – When the crown has two whirls, if the hair is cut too short it can tend to stick up where they meet.

Double wind – DUBL WIYND – A technique of winding using two perm rods per section: the first rod is wound from points to mid-length; the second rod is added and wound together with the first rod from the mid-length to the roots.

Dreadlocks – DRED-loks – A method of dressing hair into long, thin matted or tangled strands with natural or fibre hair. Also known as locking.

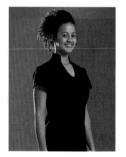

Dress code – DRESS kohd – The rules around dress/uniform, hairstyle, make-up, nails and jewellery that you are required to follow.

Dressing cream – DRESS-ing KREEM – A finishing product used to define the finished look.

Dressing out – DRESS-ing OWT – The process of brushing the hair after a set to remove all the roller marks.

Dry cutting – DRY KUT-ing – Cutting the hair while it is dry.

Dry hair – DRY HAIR – Hair that lacks moisture – it may feel rough and look dull.

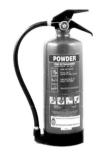

Dry powder extinguisher – DRIY POW-duh iks-TING-gwish-uh – A red fire extinguisher with a blue band, suitable for burning liquids, such as oil, paint and grease.

Dry setting – DRY SET-ing – A setting method where dry hair is wound around a roller. This does not break down the hydrogen bonds so the hair is baked into its new shape around the roller.

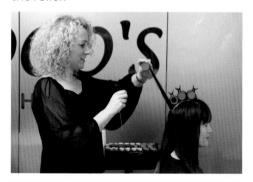

Dry shampoo – DRIY sham-POO – There are two types of dry shampoo: spirits (alcohol) and dry powders.

Dry shaving – DRY SHAY-ving – Beard shaving with an electric shaver.

Dutch braid – DUCH BRAYD – An inverted French braid – weaving the strands under rather than over creates a braid which stands out from the head, giving an 'embossed' look.

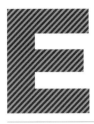

Easi meche – EE-zee MESH – Transparent wraps used for colouring specific sections of hair.

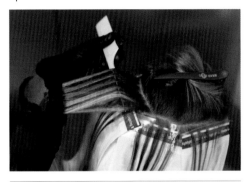

Eccrine glands – EK-rin or EK-reen or EK-riyn glandz – The major sweat glands of the human body, found in the skin. They produce a clear, odourless substance, consisting primarily of water.

Eczema – EKS-uh-muh – A non-infectious skin condition – the skin will look red and inflamed, itchy, and can split and weep. Eczema is often sore and painful, so medical referral is advisable.

Effective communication – if-FEK-tiv kuh-myoo-ni-KAY-shuhn – Giving and receiving information well, including body language, smiling and tone of voice.

Effective rapport – if-FEK-tiv ruh-POR – This means engaging in conversation with your clients so they will come back in the future and therefore create more business for your salon.

Effleurage – EF-lur-rahzh – A gentle stroking massage movement used during the shampooing and conditioning process. Used to distribute the shampoo and conditioner evenly through the hair.

Egg shampoo – EG sham-POO – Using an egg to wash your hair: the egg white is used for greasy hair and the yolk is used for dry hair.

Elasticity test – ee-lass-TISS-it-ee TEST – To determine the strength of the cortex. Hair with good elasticity will stretch and return to its original length without becoming damaged.

Electricity at work regulations – el-ek-TRISS-it-ee uht WURK reg-yuh-LAY-shuhnz – These regulations state that all electrical appliances must be tested every 12 months by a qualified electrician. It is your responsibility to ensure that you remove any defective electrical equipment, label it as faulty, report it to a responsible person and remove from use.

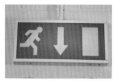

Emergency procedure

– i-MUR-juhn-see pruh-SEED-yuh – The emergency procedure is a plan of movements to evacuate a building. An emergency is a severe, often dangerous situation that needs immediate attention.

Emollient – i-MOLL-ee-uhnt – A substance used in a product to soften and enhance the appearance of the hair.

Empathy – EM-puh-thee – Understanding how another person feels and reflecting this back to the other person.

Employee – im-ploy-EE – A person who is employed by a business to do work for them.

Employee's basic rights and responsibilities – im-ploy-EEZ BAYSS-ik RIYTS uhnd ruh-sponss-i-BIL-it-eez – The law protects employees from harassment, bullying or any type of discrimination at work. Employers may be taken to court if they do not adhere to the law.

Employer – im-PLOY-uh – A person who owns a business and employs people to work for them.

Employer's liability insurance – im-PLOY-uhz ly-uh-BIL-it-ee in-SHOR-ruhnss – Employers and self-employed persons must by law hold employer's liability insurance so that they are covered if any employee suffers a body injury, illness or disease from their employment.

Employer's responsibilities – im-PLOY-uhz ruh-sponss-i-BIL-it-eez – It is the employer's responsibility to provide a safe place of work. They must put into place safety policies and procedures, as well as provide health and safety equipment and training to ensure all employees and anyone entering the salon is kept safe.

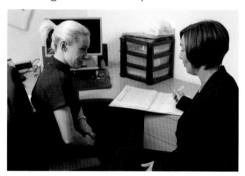

Employment Act – im-PLOY-muhnt akt – Covers the right to have statutory leave and pay for maternity/paternity.

Employment Relations Act – im-PLOY-muhnt ruh-LAY-shuhnz akt – Employees have a right to join a trade union. Part-time workers are allowed the same rights as full-time workers.

Employment tribunals – im-PLOY-muhnt try-BYOO-nuhlz – Employment tribunals deal with legal disputes in the workplace. They hear cases involving employment disputes that have not been resolved by other means.

Emulsify – i-MUL-si-fiy – A term used when removing colouring products from the hair: a small amount of water is massaged into the colour to help break down the product, enabling it to be rinsed out of the hair more easily and to avoid skin staining.

Emulsion bleach – i-MUL-shuhn BLEECH – This bleach is suitable for full head bleaches, because they have a cooling agent in them.

End paper – END PAY-puh – A resource to use when perm winding. Paper is placed around the ends of the hair to help stop buckled ends (fish hooks).

Enhancing the salon's image – in-HAHN-sing dhe SAL-o(ng)z IM-ij – Making sure the salon is attractive and appealing to the customer.

Enquiries – in-KWIY-uh-reez – Queries or requests for information from clients, with which you may deal face-to-face, over the phone or via email.

Environmental conditions – in-viy-ruhn-MENTL kuhn-DISH-uhnz – The work area must be safe and comfortable for employees and clients. Consider heating, lighting and ventilation.

Environmental factors – in-viy-ruhn-MENTL FAK-tuhz – These are the things around you in the salon. An example of a hazard caused by an environmental factor is a wet floor because it may cause someone to slip over on it.

Environmental Protection Act – in-viy-ruhn-MENTL pruh-TEK-shuhn akt – An act for waste management and control of emissions into the environment.

Environmentally damaged hair – in-viy-ruhn-MENT-uh-lee DAM-ijd HAIR – Hair that has been damaged by excessive exposure to the sun, wind, seawater or chlorine.

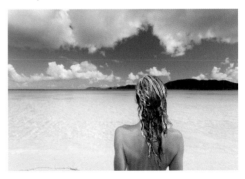

Epidermis – ep-ee-DUR-miss – The outermost layers of the skin (the visible part).

Epithelium – e-pee-THEE-lee-uhm – One of the four basic types of tissues that cover the surface of the body.

Equal opportunities – EE-kwuhl op-uh-TYOON-it-eez – By law, nobody should be discriminated against on the grounds of their age, race, gender or disability. There is legislation to enforce this, and you can see details at various websites, including www.eoc.org.uk.

Equal Pay Act – EE-kwuhl PAY akt – Employers must pay the same rate to men and women for doing the same job of equal value.

Equality – i-KWOL-it-ee – Treating people the same, regardless of differences like race or gender.

Ethical standards – ETH-ikl STAN-duhdz – This means working honestly and keeping within all the rules and regulations of your salon and the hairdressing industry.

Eumelanin – yoo-MEL-uh-nin – Natural black/brown colour pigments in the hair and skin.

Euro – YOOuh-roh – European currency.

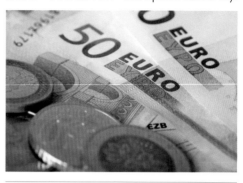

Evacuation procedure – i-vak-yoo-AY-shuhn pruh-SEED-yuh – The exit route and assembly point identified by the salon.

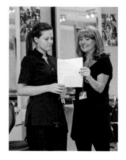

Evaluation – i-val-yoo-AY-shuhn – Actively seek feedback from a number of people (line manager, colleagues, audience, judges, models, photographer) on the impact of your image.

Evaluation methods – i-val-yoo-AY-shuhn METH-uhdz – Different ways of getting feedback – could include team meetings, or feedback from your tutor, or self-evaluation.

Evident – EV-id-uhnt – Easily seen.

Excessive moisture – ik-SESS-iv MOYSS-chuh – When the hair is too wet to carry out the next service – remove the excess moisture with a towel.

Excessive tension – ik-SESS-iv TEN-shuhn – Pulling the hair too tight when plaiting and twisting, causing traction alopecia (hair loss) at partings and around the hairline.

Exfoliation – eks-FOH-lee-AY-shuhn – Cleanses the pores of the skin, reduces skin irritation and makes shaving easier.

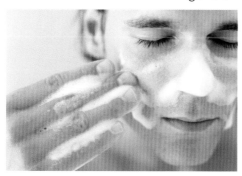

Exhibits – ig-ZIB-its – Shows.

Exothermic – eks-oh-THUR-mik – Chemical reaction that produces heat.

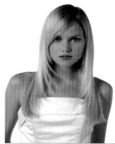

Extensions – iks-TEN-shuhnz – Adding extra hair to a hairstyle to add volume, colour and/or length.

External enquiry – eks-TUR-nuhl in-KWIY-uh-ree – A query that comes from someone outside the salon, for example a phone call from a manufacturer or client.

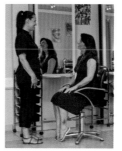

Eye contact – IY KON-takt – An effective communication tool that enables you to connect with your colleagues and clients.

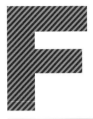

Face massage – FAYSS MASS-ahzh
– Facial massage will help to soften
the skin and distribute the lather
when shaving. You can use effleurage,
petrissage, tapotement, pinching,
friction and tapping movements on the
face during shaving services.

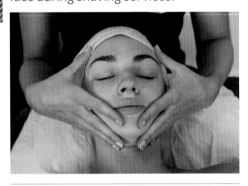

Face muscles – FAYSS MUSSLZ
– The face muscles are: frontalis,
procerus, nasalis, masseter,
zygomaticus, platysma, mentalis,
sternocleidomastoid, triangularis,
risorius, buccinators, orbicularis oris,
quadratus labii superious, orbicularis
oculi, temporalis and corrugator.

Face shape – FAYSS SHAYP – It is
important to choose a style that will
complement the face shape. There are
many facial shapes: round, oblong, oval,
square, heart, pear and rectangular.

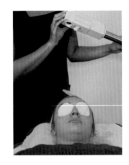

Face steamer
– FAYSS STEEM-uh
– This can be used
instead of hot
towels in facial
massage.

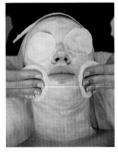

Facial – FAY-shuhl
– A skin treatment
on the face, which
may include
steam, exfoliation,
extraction, facial
masks, peels
and massage.

Facial and skull bones – FAY-shuhl
uhnd SKUL BOHNZ – The primary bones
of the face and skull are the mandible,
maxilla, zygomatic, nasal, frontal,
pariental and occipital. The point at
which bones of the skull are fused
together is called a suture.

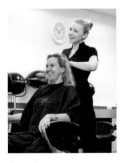

**Facial
expressions**
– FAY-shuhl
ik-SPRESH-uhnz –
Facial expressions
are a form of
non-verbal
communication.
Common
facial expressions include anger,
concentration, confusion, disgust,
excitement, empathy, fear, frustration,
glare, happiness and sadness.

Facial features – FAY-shuhl FEE-chuhz – Nose, eyes, lips, ears, high/low cheekbones and high/low forehead. These are all taken into consideration when choosing a style for the client; the style will need to complement the client's features.

Facial hair – FAY-shuhl HAIR – The facial hair tends to grow at the lip, cheeks, lower lip, chin and the rest of the lower face to form a full beard.

Facilities – fuh-SIL-it-eez – The facilities of the reception area include the seating area, cloakroom, hot and cold drinks, newspapers and magazines, and retail displays.

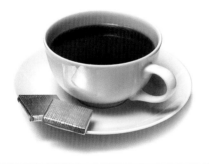

Factors – FAK-tuhz – Things to consider, such as hair condition and density, that affect your choice of product or style.

Fade – FAYD – A fade is an extreme type of taper cut, where the hair on the sides and back is cut extremely close to the head and then tapered upward.

Fashion and photographic settings – FASH-uhn uhnd foh-tuh-GRAF-ik SET-ingz – Where fashion and photographic events take place, for example fashion shows and magazine shoots.

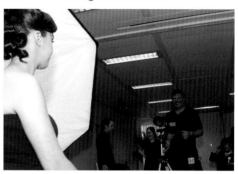

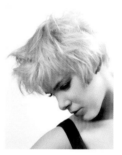

Fashion look – FASH-uhn LUUK – A style that is currently in fashion and worn for a period of time or until no longer fashionable.

Fashion trends – FASH-uhn trendz – Current popular styles in clothes, make-up, nail art, etc.

Fatigue – fuh-TEEG – Tiredness or exhaustion.

Feathering – FEDH-uh-ring – A cutting technique using the points of the scissors.

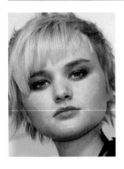

Features of the head and face
– FEE-chuhz uhv dhuh HED uhnd FAYSS – Includes nose, ears, high forehead, short forehead, chin, etc.

Features of a product – FEE-chuhz uhv uh PROD-uhkt – Use these to help you sell a product, eg clients care about the ingredients that the product contains and how it achieves a particular result.

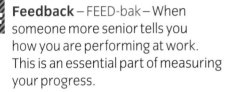

Feedback – FEED-bak – When someone more senior tells you how you are performing at work. This is an essential part of measuring your progress.

Fibrils – FIY-brilz – The microfibril is a very fine fibril, found in the hair. A microfibril is formed by 11 protofibrils; hundreds of microfibrils form a fibril; many fibrils form a cortical cell; the cortical cells are closely packed together to make up the cortex of the hair.

Financial effectiveness of the business
– fiy-NAN-shuhl i-FEK-tiv-nuhss uhv dhuh BIZ-niss – The monitoring and effective use of salon resources, and meeting productivity and development targets to make a positive contribution to the effectiveness of the business.

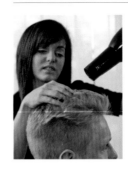

Finger drying
– FING-guh DRIY-ing – Using the fingers and hands to mould, shape and lift the hair into the required style while drying.

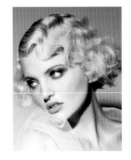

Finger waving
– FING-guh WAY-ving – A method of moulding wet hair into s-shape waves using fingers and a comb; no root lift is achieved.

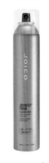

Finishing products
– FIN-ish-ing PROD-uhkts – Products used when the style has been finished to hold it in place. The products will also act as a slight barrier to any moisture with which the client may come into contact.

Finishing products – FIN-ish-ing PROD-uhkts – Used during the dressing and finishing of the style to help maintain the finished result.

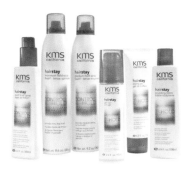

Fire evacuation – FIY-uh i-vak-yoo-AY-shuhn – The instant and speedy movement of people away from the threat of fire.

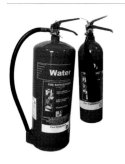

Fire extinguisher – FIY-uh iks-TING-gwish-uh – There are many different fire extinguishers, classified according to the class of fire for which they should be used. All fire extinguishers are red with a coloured band to show what type of fire it can be used for. It is very important to use the correct type of fire extinguisher.

Fire retardant – FIY-uh ruh-TAH-duhnt – A chemical used to slow down the spread of fire.

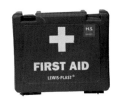

First aid – FURST AYD – First Aid is emergency treatment administered to a sick or injured person before the arrival of professional medical care. First Aid is also administered to people with minor injuries who do not need medical attention. First Aid can only be administered by a trained First Aider.

First Aid Regulations – FURST AYD reg-yuh-LAY-shuhnz – These regulations require employers to provide adequate and appropriate equipment, facilities and trained personnel to ensure their employees receive immediate attention if they are injured or taken ill at work.

Fish hooks – FISH huuks – When the ends of the hair bend back on themselves and frizz.

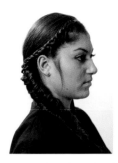

Fishtail plait
– FISH-tayl PLAT –
Also called a
herringbone plait,
this is a four-stem
plait achieved by
crossing four
pieces of the hair
over each other
to create a herringbone look, usually
in the nape area of the head.

Fixing stage – FIKS-ing STAYJ –
The neutralising stage of the perming
process, where the hydrogen is
removed from the hair by adding oxygen
(neutraliser). The disulphide bonds are
reformed into their new position.

Flammable – FLAM-uh-buhl –
Something that will burn quickly when
set alight.

Flat irons – flat IY-uhnz – More
commonly known as straightening
irons, they can be used to straighten
and flatten the hair.

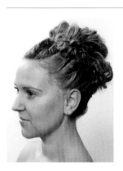

Flat twists –
FLAT TWISTS – A
method of rolling
and twisting the
hair by hand to
achieve a twist
that sits close to
the head.

Flier – FLIY-uh – Advertising leaflet for
a promotion.

Float – FLOHT – A sum of money
kept in the till to ensure the salon has
adequate change.

Foil highlighting – FOYL HIY-liy-ting
– The process of using foil to separate
strands of hair that will be lightened
from strands of hair that will remain
its natural colour.

Follicle – FOL-ikl – The cavity/opening
within the skin, from which the hairs grow.

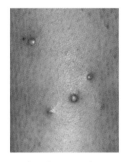

Folliculitis
– fo-lik-yuh-LIY-tiss
– A bacterial
infection of the
hair follicles,
which become
inflamed. This can
be identified by
yellow pustules
with a hair in the centre.

Fragilitas crinium – fruh-JIL-it-uhss
KRIN-ee-uhm – Commonly known as
split ends, this is when the ends of the
hair become damaged and split open.
The only real treatment for this is to
cut them off.

Fraudulent card – FRORD-yuh-luhnt
KAHD – A card that has been stolen or
is a fake.

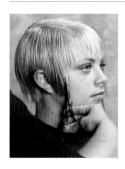

Freehand – FREE-hand – Cutting hair without holding it in place so there is no tension, for example when cutting a fringe.

Freelance – FREE-lahnss – Somebody who is self-employed and works independently.

French plait – FRENCH PLAT – This is usually a single scalp plait that involves adding sections from each side to create a smooth, neat finish.

Friction – FRIK-shuhn – A stimulating scalp massage technique applied along the path of the nerves and nerve endings on the scalp.

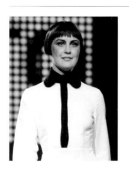

Fringe – FRINJ – Hair that covers the forehead.

Frisure forcee – frizh-YOO-uh for-SAY – The permanent curling of woven wefts.

Frizzy ends – FRIZ-ee ENDZ – This can be caused by over-processed hair, or it can be caused by fish hooks on the ends of the hair.

Frosting – FROST-ing – Colouring parts of the hair.

Full beard – FUUL BEERD – Coverage of facial hair on the upper lip, chin, sides and sideburns.

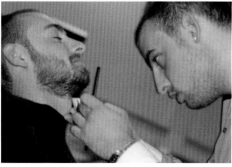

Full head application – FUUL HED ap-li-KAY-shuhn – A colouring technique that requires the colour to be applied first to the mid-lengths, then the ends, and then the roots.

Functions of the skin – FUNK-shuhnz uhv dhuh SKIN – Shapes: S = sensation; H = heat regulation; A = absorbtion; P = protection; E = excretion; S = secretion.

Fungicide – FUNG-giss-siyd – A substance that is used to kill fungi.

Fungus – FUNG-guhss – A fungus is a member of a large group of micro-organisms, many of which will cause diseases.

Furunculosis – fyuh-ruhnk-yuh-LOH-siss – An infection of the hair follicles by staphylococcal bacteria. The condition can be identified by boils and abscesses with raised, inflamed, puss-filled spots. The client will suffer irritation, swelling and pain, so this should be referred to a doctor.

Fusing – FYOO-zing – A method of attaching a strand of added hair to the natural hair using heated equipment which melts either the synthetic hair or resin.

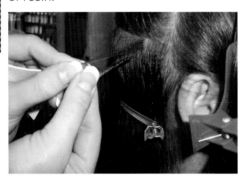

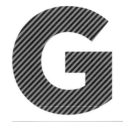

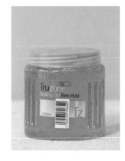

Gel – JEL – A styling product used on the hair to hold the style in place.

Gel weave – JEL WEEV – Gel is applied to wet hair and combed flat to the head; the hair is then dried and wefts of hair are bonded to this base.

Gender – JEN-duh – Whether a client is male or female.

General practitioner (GP) – JEN-ruhl prak-TISH-uh-nuh – A doctor who diagnoses illnesses and diseases, and treats patients. A GP may refer a patient on to a specialist within a particular field of medicine.

General Product Safety Regulations – JEN-ruhl PROD-uhkt SAYF-tee reg-yuh-LAY-shuhnz – This regulation relates to the safe use of all products. Follow all manufacturer's guidance and instructions when using and selling products.

Germinal matrix – JURM-in-uhl MAY-triks – An area of reproducing cells situated around the papilla at the base of the hair bulb. The germinal matrix area is where mitosis takes place and produces the keratin, which forms the three layers of the hair.

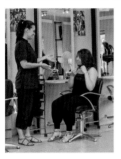

Gestures – JES-chuhz – Hand gestures are commonly used in conversations to emphasise a point.

Gift voucher – GIFT VOW-chuh – A method of payment that has already been pre-paid. The voucher can be used in full or part payment for a service.

Gloves – GLUVZ – Protective equipment to protect the hands during chemical treatments.

Glyceryl monothioglycolate – GLISS-uh-ril MON-oh-THY-oh-GLIY-koh-layt – A chemical substance used in acid perm solutions.

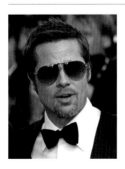

Goatee – GOH-tee – A narrow beard which arches the mouth and chin.

Goddess braids – GOD-ess braydz – A large inverted cornrow with hair added, giving the appearance of very thick hair and braids.

Goodwill and trust – guud-WIL uhnd TRUST – All solid relationships are based on this. In order to gain the goodwill and trust of your clients and colleagues, you need to show that you are friendly, helpful and dependable.

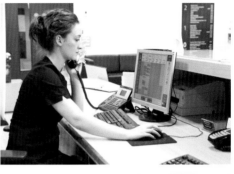

Gown – GOWN – A protective cape used to protect the client's clothing.

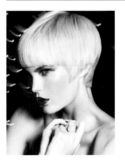

Graduating – GRAD-yoo-ay-ting – Cutting the hair to blend layers from a longer length to a shorter length, or from a shorter length to a longer length. Creative styles may include a combination of both.

Graduation – grad-yoo-AY-shuhn – A haircut with a gradual difference in length. Graduation involves cutting the hair with tension, low to medium elevation, or over direction. The final result has a layered area around the outside.

Granular layer – GRAN-yuh-luh LAY-uh – A thin layer of cells in the epidermis, also known as the stratum granulosum.

Granular pigment – GRAN-yuh-luh PIG-muhnt – The black and brown pigments found in the hair – also known as eumelanin.

Greasy hair/scalp – GREE-see HAIR/SKALP – Also known as seborrhoea, this can be caused by overactive sebaceous glands and can be identified as excessive oil on the scalp or skin.

Grey hair – GRAY HAIR – Grey hair is made up of a mixture of natural hair colour and white hair, giving a salt and pepper effect. Grey hair contains no colour pigments.

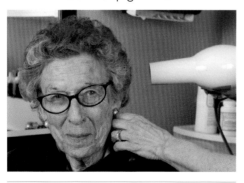

Grievance – GREE-vuhnss – Cause for complaint.

Grievance procedures – GREE-vuhnss pruh-SEED-yuhz – If you or a colleague has a dispute that can't be sorted out easily, a grievance procedure would be carried out. This would involve a formal meeting to discuss the issue. If you're unsure as to your salon's grievance procedures, ask the advice of your supervisor.

Growth cycle of the hair – GROHTH SIYKL uhv dhuh HAIR – The cycle for hair growth is anagen (growth phase), catagen (transitional phase), telogen (resting phase) and back to anagen.

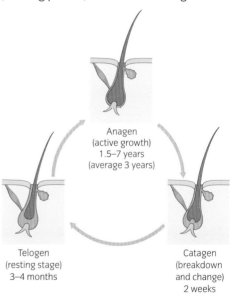

Anagen
(active growth)
1.5–7 years
(average 3 years)

Telogen
(resting stage)
3–4 months

Catagen
(breakdown
and change)
2 weeks

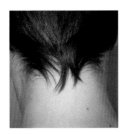

Growth patterns – GROHTH PA-tuhnz – The direction in which the hair falls. The most common growth patterns are double crown, cowlick, nape whorl and widow's peak.

Guidance – GIY-duhnss – To help, seek advice and give direction.

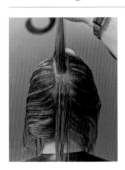

Guideline – GIYD-liyn – A cut section of hair that is used as a guide for the next section. This is sometimes known as a baseline.

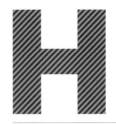

Habia – HAB-ee-ah – The Hair and Beauty Industry Authority – the government-appointed standards-setting body for hair, beauty, nails, spa therapy, barbering and African type hair. It creates the standards that form the basis of all qualifications.

Hackle – HAKL – A metal plate with rows of pointed needles used to blend or straighten hair. This tool is used as a preliminary step in the process of wig making.

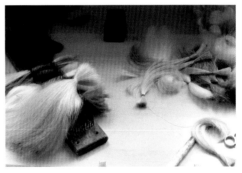

Hair analysis – HAIR uh-NAL-uh-siss – An assessment of the condition of the hair, via a visual check and manual testing, to make sure that no factors prevent a service from taking place.

Hair breakage – HAIR BRAYK-ij – Hair in poor condition; a possible cause is over-processing with chemical treatments.

G

H

Hair bulb – HAIR BULB – The root of the hair, which is whiter in colour and softer in texture than the hair shaft.

Hair condition – HAIR kuhn-DISH-uhn – The flatter the cuticles on the hair, the more light the hair will reflect, and the more the hair will give the appearance of being in better condition.

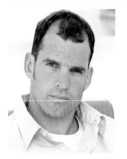

Hair density – HAIR DEN-sit-ee – The number of hairs that a person has, which will partly determine how thick a person's hair appears. Hair density can be sparse (few hairs), normal, or dense (many hairs).

Hair disorder – HAIR dis-OR-duh – A non-infectious condition of the hair which requires special consideration when carrying out hairdressing services. The service may need to be adapted for the condition of the client's hair.

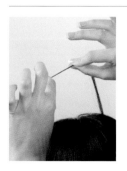

Hair elasticity – HAIR ee-lass-TISS-it-ee – The internal condition of the hair, which affects its ability to stretch and return to its original shape.

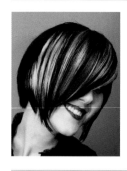

Hair extensions – HAIR ik-STEN-shuhnz – These add density, length or colour to a client's style; they can be made of synthetic or human hair.

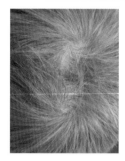

Hair growth patterns – HAIR GROHTH PAT-uhnz – This is a factor that can influence your decision as to how short to cut the hair, for example a double crown. The different types of hair growth patterns are: widow's peak, nape whorl, single/double crown and cow lick.

Hair loss – HAIR LOSS – The balding of the hair, which can be hereditary or caused by stress. Hair loss is also known as alopecia.

Hair muscle – HAIR MUSSL – The muscle attached to the hair is called an arrector pili muscle; it attaches below the gland to a fibrous layer around the outer case. When this muscle contracts, it causes the hair to stand on end, which is commonly known as goose bumps.

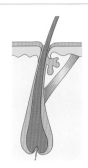

Hair papilla – HAIR puh-PIL-uh – A large structure at the base of the follicle called the papilla. The papilla is made up mainly of nerves, blood vessels and fibrous tissue.

Hair pigment – HAIR PIG-muhnt – There are two main types of pigment in the hair: eumelanin, sometimes called granular pigment (black and brown), and pheomelanin, sometimes called diffuse pigment (red and yellow).

Hair shaft – HAIR SHAHFT – The hair is made up of three layers: the cuticles, cortex and medulla.

Hair show – HAIR shoh – This could be a competition or a fashion show where hairdressers can showcase their skills.

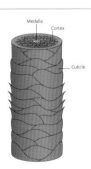

Hair structure – HAIR STRUK-chuh – The strands of hair above the skin. The hair structure has three layers, known as the cuticles, cortex and the medulla.

Hair stylist – HAIR stiyl-ist – A person who is qualified to carry out many different services within a hairdressing salon, for example cutting and hair colouring.

Hair test – HAIR TEST – Pull test, skin test, elasticity test and porosity test are all tests to determine the suitability of the service requested.

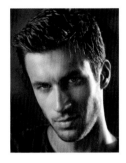

Hair texture – HAIR TEKS-chuh – The texture of the hair can be smooth or coarse. The thickness of the individual hairs can be fine, medium or coarse.

Hair threading – HAIR THRED-ing – The process of wrapping and covering the hair with coloured threads; it can also be performed on plaited hair.

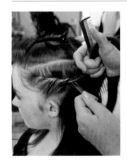

Hair twists – HAIR TWISTS – A twist that sits along the head; the hair can be continually twisted to the ends so that the twist will sit as a tuft or knot.

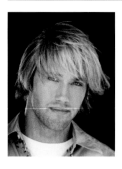

Hair type – HAIR TIYP – The client's hair type will help you to decide if the hair is too curly, wavy or straight to achieve the desired look.

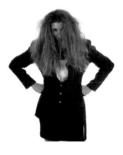

Hair types and conditions – HAIR TIYPS uhnd kuhn-DISH-uhnz – How the hair feels and looks. Types of hair are: normal, dry, oily, dandruff and damaged.

Hair wrapping – HAIR RAP-ing – Plaiting or wrapping the hair with coloured ribbons.

Hairdressing Council – HAIR-dressing KOWN-suhl – Set up in 1964 by an Act of Parliament, this industry body allows hairdressers to apply to become state registered, in the same way that doctors, dentists or nurses can.

Hairdressing organisation – HAIR-dress-ing or-guhn-iy-ZAY-shuhn – A body supporting hairdressers or regulating something in hairdressing.

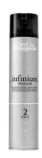

Hairspray – HAIR-spray – A finishing product used to fix the finished style in place; it helps to protect the hair from atmospheric moisture, lengthens the life of the finished style and is applied following completion of styling.

Hairstyle – HAIR-stiyl – A style that is chosen by a client.

Halitosis – hal-i-TOH-siss – A term used to describe noticeably unpleasant odours exhaled in breathing.

Hard pressing comb – HAHD PRESS-ing KOHM – Used to remove most of the curl in African hair type, but can be damaging to the hair.

Hard sell – HAHD SEL – Forceful selling technique.

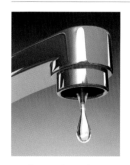

Hard water – HAHD WOR-tuh – Water with a high calcium and magnesium content, causing a poor soap and detergent interaction, which makes it hard to get the shampoo to lather and creates scum.

Harmonious working relationships
– hah-MOH-nee-uhs WUR-king
ruh-LAY-shuhn -ships – This means
working well with your colleagues and
understanding the importance of team
work. It's important, as you will work
more effectively and create a better
impression of your salon to clients.

HASAWA – AICH-AY-ESS-AY-DUBL-yoo-
AY – Standing for Health and Safety at
Work Act, it states the responsibilities
of the employer and employee. All
the other health and safety acts come
under this one.

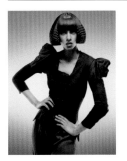

Haute coiffure
– OHT kwa-FYOO-
uh – The newest
designs from the
highest fashion.

Hazard – HAZ-uhd – Something
dangerous, with potential to cause
harm, such as scissors, chemicals,
or a trailing electric cable from a piece
of equipment.

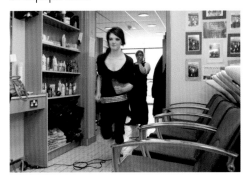

Hazardous substances – HAZ-uhd-
uhss SUB-stuhn-siz – A substance is
hazardous if it could cause harm to the
person who comes into contact with
it. For example, chemicals or cleaning
products are hazardous because if they
come into contact with the eyes or skin,
they could damage them.

Hazard symbols – HAZ-uhd SIM-
buhlz – You might see one or more
of these symbols on a single product.
They tell us if the product is toxic,
corrosive, harmful, explosive, oxidising
or flammable.

Hazardous waste – HAZ-uhd-uhss
WAYST – Waste products such as
tissues contaminated with blood.
These need to be correctly disposed
of to avoid cross-infection.

Head and face shape

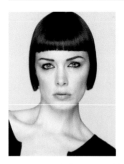

Head and face shape – HED uhnd FAYSS SHAYP – If the client chooses a style that is unsuitable for their head or face shape, it is your responsibility to offer a more suitable alternative; the ideal face shape is said to be oval.

Head and neck muscles – HED uhnd NEK MUSSLZ – Frontalis, temporalis, occipitalis, epicranial aponeurosis, sternocleidomastoid, platysma and trapezius.

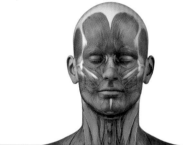

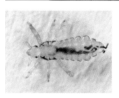

Head lice – HED LIYSS – Also known as pediculosis capitis – head lice are generally spread through direct head-to-head contact with an infested person. The symptoms are itching, red marks and scratch marks on the head. Lice feed on blood from the scalp. The egg or 'nit' may hatch one nymph that will grow and develop to an adult louse.

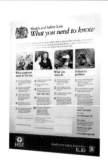

Health & Safety at Work Act (HASAWA) – HELTH uhnd SAYF-tee uht WURK akt -- AICH-AY-ESS-AY-DUBL-yoo-AY – This act states the duties of the employer and employee. All the other health and safety laws come under this one.

Health and Safety Executive – HELTH uhnd SAYF-tee ig-ZEK-yuh-tiv – The HSE's job is to prevent people being killed, injured or made ill by work.

Health and safety inspector – HELTH uhnd SAYF-tee in-SPEK-tuh – Health and safety inspectors work to protect people's health and safety, by making sure risks in the workplace are properly controlled.

Health and safety legislation – HELTH uhnd SAYF-tee lej-iss-LAY-shuhn – Laws that outline your responsibilities in protecting the health and safety of your colleagues and clients.

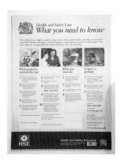

Health and safety policy – HELTH uhnd SAYF-tee POL-iss-ee – The manager of a salon is required by law to draw up a health and safety policy for their business. This must be accessible to all employees, who must read and understand the requirements of the policy.

Heat damage – HEET DAM-ij – Damage to the hair caused by excessive use of heated styling equipment, eg straighteners.

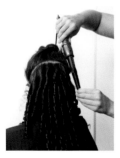

Heat moulding techniques – HEET MOHLD-ing tek-NEEKS – The process of moulding the hair with heated styling equipment, eg curling tongs, spiral wands, hot brushes and straighteners.

Heat protectors – HEET pruh-TEK-tuhz – A product that is applied to wet or dry hair to coat and protect it from damage caused by using heated styling/finishing equipment.

Heated rollers – HEET-id ROH-luhz – Rollers that are heated up and placed in dry hair to produce temporary curls in the hair.

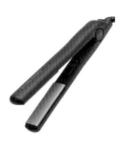

Heated styling equipment – HEET-id STIYL-ing i-KWIP-muhnt – Styling tools used to temporarily set dry hair, adding curl, volume or straightening hair; for example, straightening irons.

Heavy goods – HEV-ee GUUZ – When lifting heavy objects, you have to consider the health and safety risk. The Manual Handling Regulations are designed to protect you and minimise risks relating to the lifting and handling of heavy goods.

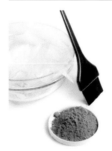

Henna – HEN-uh – A product not compatible with modern hairdressing chemical products. Compound henna contains a combination of vegetable henna and metallic salts.

Hepatitis B – hep-uh-TIY-tiss BEE – An irritation and inflammation of the liver.

Hereditary – huh-RED-it-ree – Transmitted genetically from parent to child.

Herpes simplex – HUR-peez SIM-pleks – A viral infection; the symptoms are burning, irritation, swelling and inflammation with a fluid-filled blister, usually around the lip area (commonly known as a cold sore).

Herpes zoster – HUR-peez ZOSS-tuh – A viral infection of the epidermis and nerve endings. The symptoms are painful blisters, sore and inflamed areas, and a fever. Aching and pain may continue after the condition has cleared. Affected clients should be referred to a doctor.

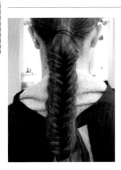

Herringbone braid – HERR-ing-bohn brayd – Often known as a fishtail plait, this is technically a four-strand braid, formed by bringing tiny sections from one half of the hair to the other.

High frequency scalp massage – HIY FREE-kwuhn-see SKALP MASS-ahzh or muh-SAHZH – A high frequency current which stimulates the surface of the scalp by means of massaging the cells of the scalp. It can also be used to stimulate local blood circulation and local glandular activity. It supplies heat and is soothing to the nervous system of the scalp.

High lift tint – HIY LITF TINT – A product that will lift and lighten the natural colour of the hair, and will also deposit tone.

Highlighting cap – HIY-liy-ting KAP – A plastic cap used to colour parts of the hair; the cap is placed onto the head and a hook is used to pull through small pieces of hair.

Highlights – HIY-liyts – A method of partially colouring the hair.

Historical eras – hiss-TORR-ikl EER-ruhz – Periods of history such as Aztec, Inca, Egyptian, Roman, Medieval or Edwardian.

HIV – AICH-IY-VEE – Human immunodeficiency virus, believed to lead to the condition AIDS.

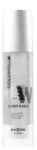

Holding gel
– HOHLD-ing jel –
A product used to achieve a firm hold on shorter looks – it can be used for finger drying, scrunching and wet looks.

Homecare and aftercare advice – HOHM-kair uhnd AHF-tuh-KAIR uhd-VIYSS – The advice given to clients to help them keep their style longer; this will include advice on maintenance of the style, tools, equipment and products.

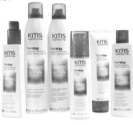

Honing – HOHN-ing – The sharpening of a razor using a stone (hone).

Hood dryer – HUUD DRIY-uh – A hairdryer used to dry hair that has been wound in setting rollers.

Hopscotch perm wind – HOP-skoch PURM wiynd – A technique used on medium to long layered hair. Three or four rods are wound to the root with weaved sections left out, which are wound in the opposite direction to sit across the top of the first rods.

Horizontal roll – ho-ri-ZON-tuhl ROHL – The hair is placed into a neat classical roll at the nape of the neck – also known as a chignon.

Horny layer – HOR-nee LAY-uh – The hard, cornified top layer of the skin, constantly being worn away and replaced by underlying tissue.

Horseshoe moustache – HOHSS-shoo muh-STAHSH – A full moustache with vertical extensions grown on the corners of the lips and down the sides of the mouth to the jaw line, resembling an upside-down horseshoe.

Hospitality – hoss-pit-AL-it-ee – This covers welcoming the client, offering refreshments and magazines, and making sure the client is comfortable.

Hot attachment methods for hair extensions – HOT uh-TACH-muhnt METH-udz fuh HAIR ik-STEN-shuhnz – These include hot bonding, pre-bonding, hot fusion and thermal bonding.

Hot brush – HOT BRUSH – A hot, round styling brush that can create curls in the hair.

Hot oil treatment – HOT OYL TREET-muhnt – Moisturising products that can be used on very dry, brittle or damaged hair.

Hot towel – HOT TOWL – Applied to the client's face before a shaving service and face massage. Steam from the towels softens the hairs and helps to lubricate the beard.

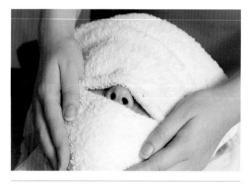

How to adapt communication – HOW tuu ah-DAPT kuh-myoo-ni-KAY-shuhn – You need to adapt your communication depending on the situation. Ways to do this are by using different tone and speed, using appropriate terminology, listening, and responding appropriately.

Human hair extensions – HYOO-muhn HAIR ik-STEN-shuhnz – Hair extensions made from human hair.

Humectants – hyoo-MEK-tuhnts – Used in skin and hair products to attract and hold moisture.

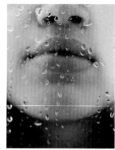

Humidity – hyoo-MID-it-ee – Moisture from the atmosphere, which may affect the condition of the hair.

Hydrogen bonds – HIY-druh-juhn BONDZ – Bonds within the hair structure; they are temporary bonds and are broken by moisture.

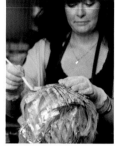

Hydrogen peroxide – HIY-druh-juhn puh-ROKS-iyd – A chemical that is mixed with permanent colour and lighteners to activate the colour.

Hydrophilic – hiy-druh-FIL-ik – Water-loving; attracted to water.

Hydrophobic – hiy-druh-FOH-bik – Water-hating; – repelled by water.

Hygiene – HIY-jeen – Cleanliness. This is extremely important in a salon, in order to work safely and get the right results.

Hygroscopic – hiy-gruh-SKOP-ik – Hair has hygroscopic properties – it is like a sponge. Something that can attract or absorb moisture from the air and is changed or altered by the absorption of moisture.

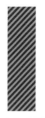

Hyperaemia – hiy-pih-REE-mee-uh – The increase of blood flow to different tissues in the body, causing a flushing of the skin.

ICT – IY-SEE-TEE – Stands for information and communication technologies, such as a smart board.

Hypersensitivity test – hiy-puh-senss-uht-IV-it-ee TEST – Also known as a skin test and patch test – used to see if the client is allergic to the product.

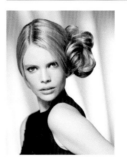

Image – IM-ij – The total look, including hair, make-up and clothes.

Hypodermis – hiy-puh-DUR-miss – A layer of tissue that lies immediately below the dermis of the skin.

Immune system – i-MYOON SISS-tuhm – The body's defence against infectious micro-organisms, including bacteria, fungi and viruses.

Impetigo – im-pi-TIY-goh – Caused by a bacterial infection, pustules become crusted and are highly contagious – medical referral should be given.

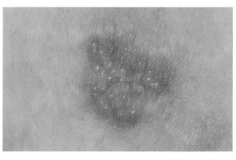

Implication – im-pli-KAY-shuhn – A likely effect or consequence.

Incentives – in-SEN-tivz – Rewards that you get when you've reached your target, which will give you the motivation to work towards them.

Incompatibility – in-kuhm-pat-uh-BIL-it-ee – When a previous service or product is present in the hair and will cause a reaction with any chemicals added to the hair.

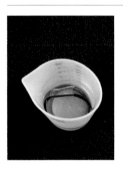

Incompatibility test – in-kuhm-pat-uh-BIL-it-ee TEST – A test carried out before colouring and perming to show whether there are chemicals present in the hair that contain metallic salts.

Incompatible – in-kuhm-PAT-uhbl – Unsuitable.

Indigo – IN-di-goh – A natural dye extracted from the leaves of plants; it has a distinctive blue–black colour.

Industry – IN-duh-stree – A type of organised activity that generates money, for example ladies' hairdressing or barbering.

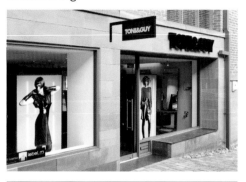

Industry sector – IN-duh-stree SEK-tuh – A group of similar industries. For example, hair and beauty is an industry sector.

Infection of the skin – in-FEK-shuhn uhv dhuh SKIN – The growth of micro-organisms caused by bacteria, viruses or fungi. A condition that may cause visible signs of swelling, or redness on the skin, and may spread.

Infectious condition – in-FEK-shuhss kuhn-DISH-uhn – The spreading from one person to another.

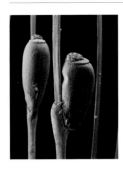

Infestation
– in-fess-TAY-shuhn – When animal parasites, such as head lice, move to a person's head and body, and then live off the nutrients found in the skin, blood and tissue.

Infill colour – IN-fil KUH-luh – A colour that is placed in-between foils, mesh or wraps. This is ideal for a client who has a high percentage of white but still likes a combination of colours.

Inflammation – in-fluh-MAY-shuhn – A condition in which the affected part of the body becomes hot, swollen and sometimes painful.

Influencing factors – IN-floo-uhn-sing FAK-tuhz – You must consider certain factors before and during the hairdressing service. These may include existing colour, previous services, and the condition of the hair and scalp.

Influenza – in-floo-EN-zuh – Commonly referred to as the flu, the most common symptoms are change in body temperature, coughing, sore throat and headache.

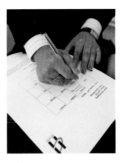

Information
required – in-fuh-MAY-shuhn ruh-KWIY-uhd – When making an appointment, the receptionist must record the following information: customer's name and contact details, service or treatment required, time of appointment date of appointment and the name of the person who will provide the service or treatment.

Infrared lamp – IN-fruh-RED LAMP – An accelerator that uses infrared heat as a source of heat to speed up the service.

Ingrowing hair – IN-groh-ing HAIR – When hair growing in the follicle becomes trapped underneath the skin's surface and grows back into the skin, causing irritation.

Inhaling – in-HAY-ling – Breathing in.

Instructional techniques – in-STRUK-shuhn-uhl tek-NEEKS – Used to present and instruct information, eg skills demonstrations, diagrams, written instructions, verbal explanations.

Instructions – in-STRUK-shuhnz – A detailed description of how to carry out a service or how to use a product.

Insurance – in-SHOH-ruhnss – Protection for you and your business; this can include public liability insurance, professional indemnity insurance and employer's liability.

Internal enquiry – in-TUR-nuhl in-KWIY-uh-ree – A question that comes from someone inside the salon, for example a client enquiring about appointment availability.

Internal verification – in-TUR-nuhl verr-i-fi-KAY-shuhn – This a system of quality checks made by someone in the centre to ensure that assignments have been written correctly and that assessment decisions are accurate. It is a recorded discussion between two professionals to ensure accuracy, fairness, consistency and quality of assessment. It does not involve the learner.

International colour chart – in-tuh-NASH-nuhl KUH-luh chaht – A chart showing all the colours in the range for specific colouring manufacturers. The basic hair colours range from one to ten, with ten being the lightest.

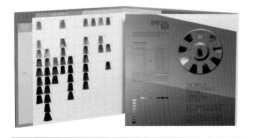

Invalid card – in-VAL-id KAHD – A card that has expired or has been refused due to lack of funds in the client's bank account or because the client has exceeded their credit limit.

Invalid currency – in-VAL-id KURR-uhn-see – Currency from another country, or old versions of coins and notes, that cannot be used.

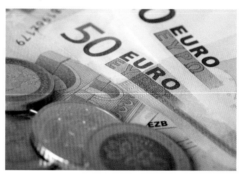

Inventory – IN-vuhn-tree or in-VENT-uh-ree – A list of the goods you have in stock.

Involuntary muscle – in-VOL-uhn-tree MUSSL – Any muscle that you can't consciously control, such as the heart.

Irritant contact dermatitis – IRR-it-uhnt KON-takt dur-muh-TIY-tiss – This skin condition can develop at any time. The symptoms are dryness, redness, itching, flaking/scaling, cracking/blistering and pain. You can help to prevent contracting dermatitis by wearing non-latex disposable gloves when using any colouring product.

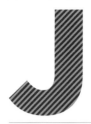

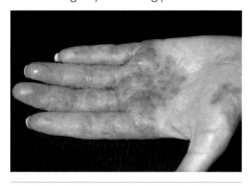

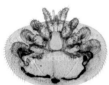

Itch mite – ICH miyt – An animal parasite that causes scabies.

Job description – JOB di-SKRIP-shuhn – This is a list of the general duties of a role. It may often include the position to which the employee reports, and specifications such as the qualifications or skills needed by the person in the job.

Job responsibilities – JOB ruh-spon-suh-BIL-it-eez – A detailed list of all the jobs you will be required to undertake.

Job roles – JOB ROHLZ – The tasks and responsibilities that each person in the workplace is there to carry out.

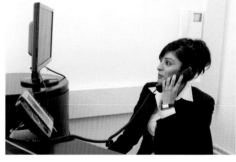

Jockey clip – JOK-ee KLIP – Used on the silks in weaving to prevent the end knot loosening.

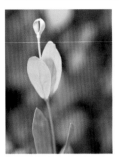

Jojoba – HOH-HOH-buh or huh-HOH-buh – Produced from a desert plant called simmondsia chinensis, its oil is an effective conditioner, moisturiser, cleanser and softener for the skin and hair. Jojoba shampoo is ideal for normal to dry hair types.

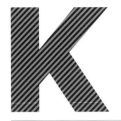

Kanekalon – kuh-NEK-uh-lon – A synthetic hair used in extensions and added hair.

Keloids – KEE-loydz – Keloids are the excess growth of scar tissue at the site of a healed skin injury; they are not medically dangerous, but they may affect the appearance.

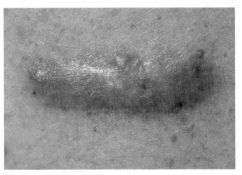

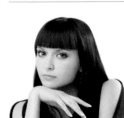

Keratin – KERR-uh-tin – The principle protein of the hair, skin and nails.

Knots – NOTS – Twisting the hair until it recoils on itself to produce a knot.

Knotting – NOT-ing – The point of intertwining and tying of hairs to a net or gauze foundation.

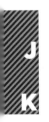

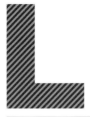

Lacklustre – LAK-luh-stuh – Drab and dull.

Lacquer – LAK-uh – A product that is sprayed onto hair to keep it in style – also known as hairspray. The spray can be dispensed from a pump or aerosol spray.

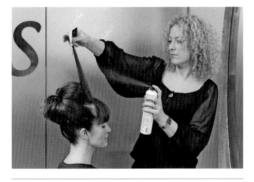

Lactic acid – LAK-tik ASS-id – A common ingredient found in surface conditioner.

Lanolin – LAN-uh-lin – A common ingredient found in surface conditioner.

Lanthionine bond – lan-thee-OH-neen BOND – During the relaxing process, the sodium hydroxide relaxer forms a new bond called a lanthionine bond.

Lanugo hair – luh-NYOO-goh HAIR – These are the fine hairs found on the foetus. They are normally shed before birth and replaced by vellus hair.

Lather – LAH-dhuh or LA-dhuh – A product applied before shaving to help cleanse the beard and lubricate the skin, allowing the razor to glide more easily.

Layers – LAY-uhz – The three layers of the hair are like a pencil. The cuticle is like the varnish on the outside of a pencil, which sometimes gets a little flaky. The cortex is like the wood in the pencil, giving it strength, and the medulla is like the lead.

Lecithin – LESS-i-thin – A common ingredient in a surface conditioner.

Legal requirements – LEE-guhl ruh-KWIY-uh-muhnts – You need to know the laws relating to health and safety, data protection, equal opportunities and disability discrimination.

Legal tender – LEE-guhl TEN-duh – Money that is legal in a given country.

Legislation – lej-iss-LAY-shuhn – Laws which must be adhered to, such as health and safety legislation.

Lemon juice – LEM-uhn JOOSS – Contains citric acid, which will remove soap scum.

Lethargy – LETH-uh-jee – A feeling of tiredness and indifference.

Lifestyle – LIYF-stiyl – Any aspects of a client's life, such as job, hobbies and family situation, that need to be considered when completing a consultation with a client.

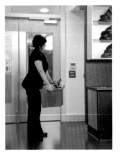

Lifting objects – LIFT-ing OB-jekts – When lifting heavy objects, you have to consider the health and safety risk. The Manual Handling Regulations are designed to protect you and minimise risks relating to the lifting and handling of heavy goods.

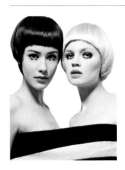

Lightener – LIYT-uh-nuh – Products that lighten the natural pigments of the hair without depositing artificial colour, otherwise known as bleach or pre-lighteners.

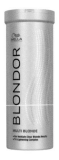

Lightening products – LIYT-uh-ning PROD-uhkts – These are products that lighten the hair, such as bleach.

Limescale – LIYM-skayl – This is the hard, off-white, chalky deposit, calcium carbonate found in the bottom of kettles.

Limited company – LIM-it-id KUM-puh-nee – A company that has shareholders.

Limits of authority – LIM-its uhv orth-ORR-it-ee – This describes work that you are not allowed to do in your salon, such as dealing with refunds on reception. You must refer these to a senior team member.

Line manager – LIYN MAN-i-juh – The manager to whom you report directly.

Linear patterns – LIN-ee-uh PAT-uhnz – Patterns created on the head; they can be straight, curved or a combination of both.

Link-selling – LINK-SEL-ing – The recommendation of products and services to meet a client's needs and enhance their experience.

Litigation – liti-GAY-shuhn – Legal action.

Litmus paper – LIT-muhss PAY-puh – The main use of litmus paper is to test whether a solution is acidic or alkaline.

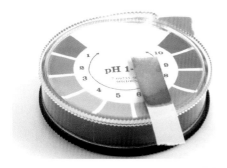

Local by-law – LOH-kuhl BY-LOH – A local council rule.

Local Government (Miscellaneous Provisions) Act 1982 – LOH-kuhl GUV-uhn-muhnt (miss-uh-LAY-nee-uhss pruh-VIZH-uhnz) akt NIYN-teen AY-tee-TOO – This requires salons performing cosmetic skin piercing such as ear piercing to register with their local authority.

Locking – LOK-ing – A styling technique generally used on African hair.

Locking stages – LOK-ing STAY-jiz – The budding stage, the growing stage and the mature stage.

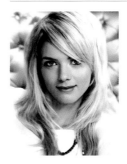

Long graduation – LONG grad-yoo-AY-shuhn – The inner layers of the hair lengths are shorter than the outline shape.

Longevity – lon-JEV-uh-tee – Longer lasting.

Loss of depth – LOSS uhv DEPTH – This is where a colour has faded by one or more shades.

Lowlighting – LOH-liy-ting – Colouring parts of the hair with a darker colour to enhance the style.

Lye-based relaxer – LIY-BAYST ri-LAKS-uh – The main active ingredient in a lye-based relaxer is sodium hydroxide. The pH level is higher in a lye relaxer than a no-lye relaxer (approximately 12–14 for lye, and 9–11 for no-lye).

Lubricant – LOO-brik-uhnt – A product that contains oils, making the external surface of the skin feel greasy and slippery.

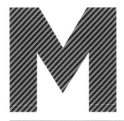

Macrofibrils – mak-roh-FIY-brilz – Microfibrils twist together to form macrofibrils. These are the fibres that make up the cells in the cortex in the hair.

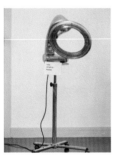

Maintenance – MAYN-tuh-nuhnss – The repair and overhaul of tools and equipment. It also includes performing routine checks to keep the equipment in safe working order and fully functional.

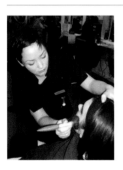

Make-up artist – MAYK-uhp AH-tist – A person who applies make-up for a variety of occasions in various settings, for example in a department store or on a fashion shoot.

Male pattern baldness – MAYL PAT-uhn BORLD-nuhss – Also known as hereditary alopecia and androgenic alopecia, it generally starts with thinning of the hair around the front hairline and on the crown area of the head.

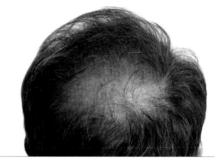

Man-made extensions – MAN-MAYD iks-TEN-shuhnz – Hair extensions made from synthetic/acrylic fibre.

Management – MAN-ij-muhnt – The act of getting people together to achieve desired goals using available resources efficiently and effectively.

Mandible – MAN-dib-uhl – The mandible is the lower jaw or jawbone.

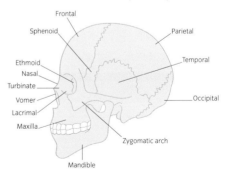

Frontal
Sphenoid
Parietal
Ethmoid
Nasal
Temporal
Turbinate
Vomer
Lacrimal
Occipital
Maxilla
Zygomatic arch
Mandible

Manipulate – muh-NIP-yuh-layt – Handle skilfully.

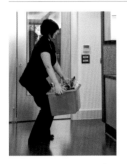

Manual Handling Operations Regulations – MAN-yoo-uhl HAND-ling op-uh-RAY-shuhnz reg-yuh-LAY-shuhnz – These regulations are designed to protect you by minimising risks relating to the lifting and handling of heavy goods.

Manufacturer's instructions – man-yuh-FAK-chuh-ruhz in-STRUK-shuhnz – Guidance by manufacturers or suppliers on the use of products, tools and equipment.

Marcel waving – MAH-SEL WAYV-ing – Finger waves are similar to the Marcel wave in appearance. The main difference is that the Marcel wave is achieved by heated curling irons.

Market research – MAH-kit ruh-SURCH – The collection and analysis of data about a particular target market and competitors in that market.

Marteau weft – MAH-TOH WEFT – A postiche made with flat sewn weft, with two loops at each end, by which it can be secured using pins or grips. The weft can be mounted onto a hair slide, hair comb or postiche clip.

Massage – MASS-ahzh or muh-SAHZH – The manipulation of the muscle and connective tissue to enhance function, aid the healing process, and promote relaxation and well-being.

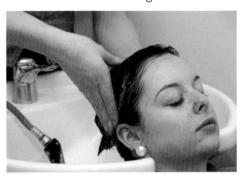

Massage media – MASS-ahzh MEE-dee-uh or muh-SAHZH MEE-dee-uh – This is the use of pre-blended oils, treatment conditioners, treatment shampoos and spirit based when performing massage services for clients.

Massage techniques – MASS-ahzh tek-NEEKS or muh-SAHZH tek-NEEKS – The different types of massage available in the salon, such as effleurage, friction, rotary and petrissage.

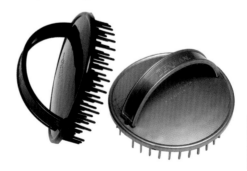

Materials, tools and equipment
– muh-TEER-ee-uhlz TOOLZ uhnd i-KWIP-muhnt – Materials include products such as perm lotion and shampoo. Tools include hand-held kit such as scissors, combs and brushes. Equipment includes electrical equipment such as dryers and accelerators.

Maternity leave – muh-TUR-nit-ee LEEV – As an employee, you have the right to 26 weeks of Ordinary Maternity Leave and 26 weeks of Additional Maternity Leave, making one year in total. The combined 52 weeks is known as Statutory Maternity Leave.

Maxilla – mak-SIL-uh – The maxilla is a fusion of two bones along the palatal fissure that form the upper jaw.

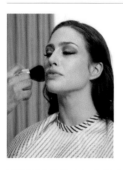

Media – MEE-dee-uh – Make-up, accessories, ornamentation, clothes, etc.

Medical referral – MED-ikl ruh-FURR-uhl – Referring a particular hair, skin or scalp condition to a specialist to investigate the problem. The referrals should be made to a general practitioner, dermatologist, pharmacist or a trichologist.

Medicated shampoo – ME-di-kay-tid sham-POO – This shampoo is particularly suitable for those with easily irritated and sensitive scalps. It contains antiseptics, such as juniper and tea tree oil, and will help to maintain a healthy hair and scalp.

Medication – me-di-KAY-shuhn – Treatment with drugs.

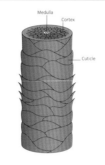

Medulla

Cortex

Cuticle

Medulla – me-DUL-uh – This is the middle section of the hair and is not affected by hairdressing treatments.

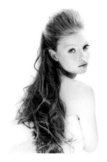

Melanin – MEL-uh-nin – The pigment that gives colour to the skin and hair. Different types of melanin give hair different colours; for example, eumelanin is responsible for black and brown tones and pheomelanin is responsible for the red and yellow tones.

Merchandise – MUR-chuhn-dyz – Goods for sale, such as shampoos, hair brushes, etc.

Mesh – MESH – A packet used for highlighting and slicing techniques.

Metallic dyes – muh-TAL-ik DIYZ – Metallic dyes are also known as inorganic dyes; they contain metallic salts. These dyes are not compatible with hydrogen peroxide.

Metallic salts – muh-TAL-ik SOLTS – Can be found in some home products which contain lead compounds or a variety of other metals, depending on the shade of colour required. These products are not compatible with salon professional products.

Methods of communication – METH-uhdz uhv kuh-myoo-ni-KAY-shuhn – Your communication with clients may be face-to-face, by letter, fax, phone, email, internet, intranet or any other method you would be expected to use within your job role.

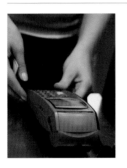

Methods of payment – METH-uhdz uhv PAY-muhnt – The different ways payments can be made, for example cash, voucher, cheque and debit card.

Methods of sterilisation – METH-uhdz uhv sterr-il-iy-ZAY-shuhn – The most reliable methods are dry heat and steam sterilising, but other methods are ultraviolet and chemical. You must use these to remove any germs from your tools and equipment.

Micro-organisms – miy-kroh-OR-guhn-iz-uhmz – Tiny living beings; they include bacteria, fungi and viruses.

Microfibrils – miy-kroh-FIY-brilz – Cross-link polypeptide chains called helix coils twist together like a piece of rope to form microfibrils in the cortex.

Minimum wage – MIN-i-muhm WAYJ – The National Minimum Wage (NMW) is a minimum amount per hour that workers in the UK are entitled to be paid.

Mint shampoo – MINT sham-POO – Cooling mint revives normal to oily hair, helping to cleanse the scalp.

Mitosis – miy-TOH-siss – Cell division.

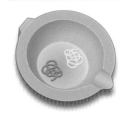

Mixing ratio – MIKS-ing RAY-shee-oh – The relative amounts of each component of a mixture; for example, quasi-permanent colours are mixed at a 1:2 ratio of colour to developer.

Moisturiser – MOYSS-chuh-riy-zuh – A styling product used to add moisture to hair; this can be applied prior to or following drying.

Moisturising balm – MOYSS-chuh-riy-zing BAHM – A product used to control unruly hair. Use on damp hair, distributing evenly throughout the hair.

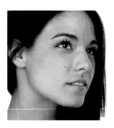

Moles – MOHLZ – Moles are usually a brownish colour, although some may be darker or skin-coloured. They can be flat or raised, smooth or rough; some have hairs growing from them.

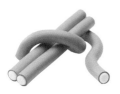

Molten brown curlers – MOHL-tuhn BROWN KUR-luhz – Long bendy rollers used for spiral curling.

Mongoloid hair – MONG-guh-loyd HAIR – Asian hair – lank and straight.

Monilethrix – muh-NIL-uh-THRIKS – A condition caused by irregular development of the hair when it is forming in the hair follicle (beaded hair). The symptoms are bead-like swelling of the hair and breakage close to the skin. Conditioning may help; otherwise, refer to a doctor.

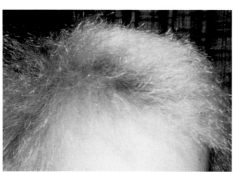

Mood board – MOOD bord – A type of poster that consists of colours, images, text, samples of materials, etc. You will produce a mood board to help develop your image concept and to communicate the concept to others.

Moulding cream – MOHLD-ing KREEM – A product used to style and finish the hair with a firm hold.

Moulding stage – MOHLD-ing stayj – A stage in the perming process when the hair has been softened and takes up the shape of the rod.

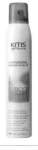

Mousse – MOOSS – A styling product used in blow drying and setting to lengthen the life of the finished style.

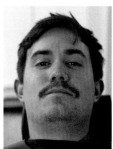

Moustache – muh-STAHSH – Facial hair that is grown on the surface above the top lip.

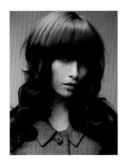

Movement
– MOOV-muhnt
– When the hair displays volume, curl or waves.

Muscles of the face, head and neck
– MUSSLZ uhv dhuh FAYSS HED uhnd NEK – The muscles are frontalis, levator labatis, zygomaticus minor, zygomaticus major, masseter, triangularis, depressor labii, sternocleidomastoid, trapezius, temporalis, procerus, corrugator, orbicularis oculi, orbicularis oris, buccinator, risorius, mentalis, platysma.

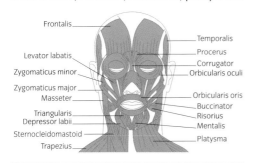

Musculoskeletal disorders
– MUSK-yuh-loh-SKEL-itl diss-OR-duhz – Muscle and bone disorders.

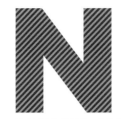

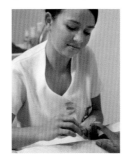

Nail technician
– NAYL tek-NISH-uhn – A person who can carry out a variety of nail services, for example manicures or nail enhancements.

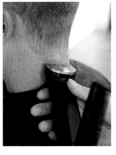

Nape
– NAYP – The back of the neck.

Nape whorl
– NAYP WURL or WORL or HWURL or HWORL – A hair growth pattern, where the hair at the nape grows in a circular pattern.

National Occupational Standards
– NASH-nuhl ok-yuh-PAY-shuhn-uhl STAN-duhdz – The Hairdressing and Beauty Therapy Industry Authority (Habia) writes the standards for the hairdressing and beauty therapy industries. Your NVQ/SVQ is based on standards written by Habia and you can read these to check what you need to be competent at in order to achieve your Level 2 NVQ/SVQ.

National Vocational Qualification (NVQ) – NASH-nuhl vuh-KAY-shuhn-uhl kwol-if-i-KAY-shuhn – A 'competence-based' qualification: this means you carry out practical, work-related tasks designed to help you develop the skills and knowledge to do a job effectively.

Natural colour – NACH-ruhl KUH-luh – A client's own colour produced from melanin.

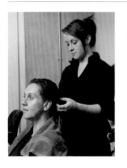

Natural fall
– NACH-ruhl FORL – When the hair is wet you can see how the hair lies: does it fall to one side or the other? Is there a natural parting?

Natural hair – NACH-ruhl HAIR – Hair that has not been chemically treated. Also known as virgin hair.

Natural parting – NACH-ruhl PAH-ting – The natural fall of the hair.

Natural pigmentation – NACH-ruhl pig-men-TAY-shuhn – The hair's natural consistency of eumelanin and pheomelanin.

Necessary actions – NESS-uh-serr-i AK-shuhnz – When a client is not suitable for the treatment and therefore it cannot be carried out, they would need to seek medical advice. In some instances the treatment could be modified.

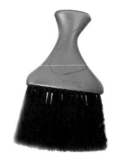

Neck brush
– NEK BRUSH – A brush designed to remove unwanted excess hair from the client's skin around the neck area, to help with client comfort.

Neckline shapes – NEK-liyn SHAYPS – It is always best to follow the natural growth pattern of the hairline. This could be rounded, square or tapered.

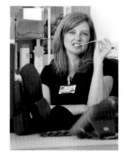

Negative behaviour
– NEG-uh-tiv bi-HAYV-ee-uh – This is bad behaviour while working in the salon, for example offensive body language, poor/rude attitude or unprofessional personal presentation.

Neutral – NYOO-truhl – Neither acid nor alkaline, with a pH close to 7.

Neutralise – NYOO-truh-liyz – The process of reconditioning or rebalancing the hair. From this process, the hair is returned to its natural state of pH 4.5–5.5.

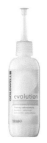

Neutraliser – NYOO-truh-liyz-uh – An ingredient that stabilises the hair structure, hardening the hair to take the shape of the perm rod.

Neutralising – NYOO-truh-liyz-ing – A chemical process used to fix the hair in a new position after it has been altered by the action of the perm lotion.

Neutralising shampoo – NYOO-truh-liyz-ing sham-POO – Used to cleanse the hair of any remaining relaxer and neutralise any alkalinity still present.

Neutralising tones – NYOO-truh-liyz-ing TOHNZ – Correcting an unwanted tone in the hair by introducing the opposite colour to cancel it out; for example, green tones are neutralised by red.

New clients – NYOO KLIY-uhnts – Clients that are new to the salon.

Nine-section perm wind – NIYN-SEK-shuhn PURM WIYND – A sectioning technique where the hair is divided into nine sections, using clips to secure the hair. This can be done prior to winding the hair, making the hair easier to control.

Nitro dyes – NIY-troh DIYZ – These are semi-permanent colours, with large and small molecules. They sit just below the cuticles on the outer edge of the cortex.

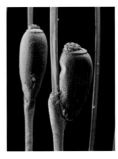

Nits – NITS – Also known as pediculosis capitis and head lice; the lice are generally spread through direct head contact with an infested person. The symptoms are itching, red marks and scratch marks on the head. Lice feed on blood from the scalp.

No-lye relaxer – NOH-LIY ri-LAKS-uh – These relaxers contain calcium hydroxide and are less irritating on the scalp, causing less itching and burning during the relaxing process.

Non-conventional – NON-kuhn-VEN-shuhn-uhl – Something not normally used, for example setting hair on chopsticks or pipe cleaners.

Non-infectious skin condition – NON-in-FEK-shuhss SKIN kun-DISH-uhn – A condition that does not spread from one person to another, for example eczema.

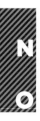

Non-verbal communication

Non-verbal communication – non-VUR-buhl kuh-myoo-ni-KAY-shuhn – Communicating without speaking, for example via written-down notes and messages, listening, nodding, smiling, eye contact, frowning and sign language.

Normal hair – NORM-uhl HAIR – Hair that is neither too dry nor too greasy.

Normaliser – NORM-uh-liyz-uh – Also known as neutraliser.

Normalising products – NORM-uh-liyz-ing PROD-uhkts – Post-relaxing products used as neutralising products after the relaxing process.

Notched scissors – NOCHT SIZ-uhz – These are a form of thinning scissors; they are also known as serrated scissors and thinning scissors.

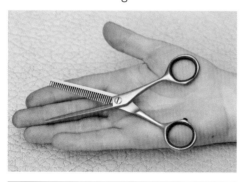

Nozzle – NOZL – The end of a hairdryer, used for directing the air flow.

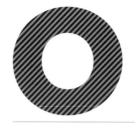

Objection/overcoming objections – uhb-JEK-shun/oh-vuh-KUM-ing uhb-JEK-shuhnz – An objection can be seen as the client putting up resistance to buying the product. A good sales person will be able to recognise if the objection is valid, and so close the discussion, or if the client just needs reassurance, in which case they will convince the client that they are doing the right thing by buying it.

Objective – uhb-JEK-tiv – A goal to reach; for example, the salon may have identified the need to take an agreed total amount of money each week in retail sales.

Observation – ob-zuh-VAY-shuhn – To watch and receive knowledge information on what someone is achieving.

Obstruction – uhb-STRUK-shuhn – An item in the way of where you wish to get to, eg a blocked emergency door.

Occasion – uh-KAY-zhuhn – A special event (such as a wedding or party) for which clients often have their hair styled. You will create appropriate styles for these.

Occipital bone – ok-SIP-it-uhl BOHN – The bone across the back of the head above the nape area.

Occipitofrontalis muscle – ok-SIP-i-toh-fron-TAH-liss MUSSL – A muscle which covers parts of the skull – also known as epicranius.

Occupational role – ok-yuh-PAY-shuhn-uhl ROHL – The activities that a person is employed to carry out as part of their job.

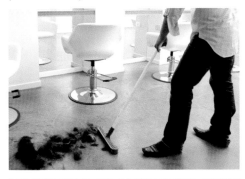

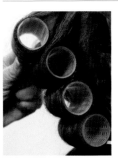

Off base – OFF BAYSS – A style of setting hair which provides no volume at the roots.

Oil bleach – OYL BLEECH – An oil-based bleach that is mixed with peroxide and a booster packet.

Oil conditioner – OYL kuhn-DISH-uh-nuh – Conditioners that contain olive oil, almond oil, coconut oil or pure vegetable oil; they can be applied to dry hair and put under heat to help penetrate into the hair.

Oils – OYLZ – Also called serums, these help to protect the hair prior to straightening or tonging. They add gloss to the hair, replace lost moisture in dry hair and are applied following completion of styling.

Oily hair – OY-lee HAIR – Hair that has an excess of sebum (the hair's natural oil). It may look lank and feel oily.

On base – ON BAYSS – A style of setting hair that creates volume at the roots. This is achieved by the roller sitting on its own base.

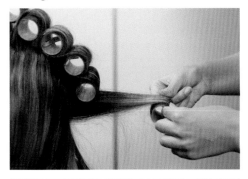

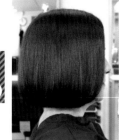

One-length cut – WUN-LENGTH KUT – The hair is cut to the same outside length around the head.

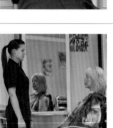

Open questions – OH-puhn KWES-chuhnz – Questions requiring full answers, rather than yes or no answers. They help to keep the conversation flowing during a consultation.

Open razor – OH-puhn RAY-zuh – A cut-throat razor that can be used to remove bulk and length.

Optional unit – OP-shuhn-uhl YOO-nit – Units that can be chosen by the candidate depending on their career direction.

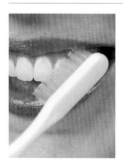

Oral hygiene – OR-uhl HIY-jeen – Regular cleaning of the teeth to ensure fresh breath and to prevent tooth decay.

Orbicularis oculi muscle – or-bik-yoo-LA-riss OK-yoo-lee (or OK-yoo-liy) MUSSL – The muscle in the face that closes the eyelids.

Orbicularis oris muscle – or-bik-yoo-LA-riss OR-iss MUSSL – A complex of muscles around the lips and mouth.

Organisational requirements – or-guhn-iy-ZAY-shuhn-uhl ruh-KWIY-uh-muhnts – Working practices and conditions specified by the salon.

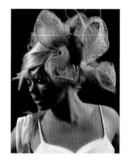

Ornamentation – or-nuh-men-TAY-shuhn – An object used to complement a style, which adds interest and detail to the finished look.

Outlines – OWT-lynz – The perimeter of the haircut, beard, moustache or sideburn shape.

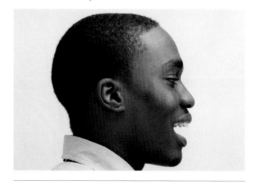

Ova – OH-vuh – The eggs of a head louse.

Over-bleaching – OH-vuh-BLEECH-ing – When a bleach application is applied over a previous application.

Over-booking – OH-vuh-BUUK-ing – Booking too many clients in at the same time, when there is not enough staff to complete the services.

Over processed – OH-vuh PROH-sesst – Over-processed hair is hair that is damaged by the excessive use of chemicals. This may cause hair breakage.

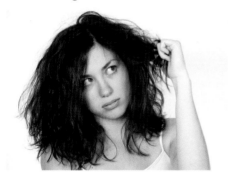

Overlapping – OH-vuh-LAP-ing – When a product is applied to previously relaxed treated hair. This will weaken the hair and eventually result in breakage or, in the case of overlapping of two colours, it can cause darker bands. Colour on colour goes darker.

Oxidant – OKS-id-uhnt – An oxidising agent such as hydrogen peroxide.

Oxidation – oks-id-AY-shuhn – A reaction caused by introducing oxygen to another chemical, for example, mixing hydrogen peroxide with lightening products (powder bleach).

Oxidation perming process – ok-si-DAY-shuhn PURM-ing PROH-sess – This takes place during the neutralising stage, when oxygen is added to the process.

Oxidation tints – ok-si-DAY-shuhn TINTS – When hydrogen peroxide is added to the tint and mixed together.

Oxidising agent – OKS-id-iyz-ing AY-juhnt – Either hydrogen peroxide or sodium bromate – a substance that allows oxidisation.

Oxymelanin – OKS-ee-MEL-uh-nin – A colourless molecule.

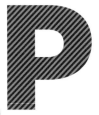

Papilla – puh-PIL-uh – This is where the hair source starts to grow; blood vessels bring food and oxygen to the papilla.

Para – PARR-uh – Short for paraphenylenediamine.

Paraphenylenediamine – parr-uh-FEN-uh-leen-DIY-uh-meen – An ingredient of many hair colours, sometimes causing an allergic reaction.

Parasite – PARR-uh-SIYT – An organism that lives in close relationship with another organism, causing it harm. For example, viruses are common parasites. The parasite has to be in its host to live, grow and multiply.

Partial head – PAH-shuhl HED – A service that is applied to a specific part of the head, eg a block colour or T section.

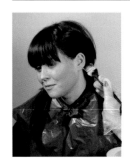

Patch test – PACH TEST – This is also known as a skin test and a hypersensitivity test; it is performed to check for allergic reactions to colouring products.

Pathogens – PATH-uh-juhnz – Also known as an infectious agent or germ, it is an agent that causes damage to its host. There are different types, for example viral, bacterial and fungal. Bacteria that cause disease are called pathogenic bacteria.

Payment card – PAY-muhnt KAHD – This refers to a debit or credit card.

Payment discrepancies – PAY-muhnt diss-KREP-uhn-siz – When there is a problem with a payment. Reasons for this may be an invalid credit/debit card or if you suspect that the card is fraudulent, or incorrect change is given.

Payment dispute – PAY-muhnt diss-PYOOT – When there is a problem with a payment, for example an invalid debit/credit card, or if you suspect the card is fraudulent.

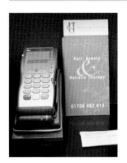

Payment methods – PAY-muhnt METH-uhdz – These may include cash, credit/debit cards, cheque or cash alternatives (for example, vouchers).

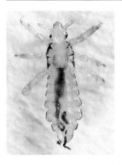

Pediculosis capitis – pi-dik-yuh-LOH-siss kuh-PIY-tiss – This condition is caused by an infestation of the head by lice. The head louse attacks the skin and feeds by puncturing the skin to suck the blood; it lays eggs (ova) on the hair close to the skin. The symptoms are an itchy scalp and red areas; you should be recommend treatment by a doctor or products from a chemist.

Peer – PEER – One of the same rank or position.

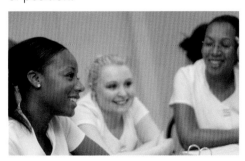

Peer assessment – PEER uh-SESS-muhnt – When a student's work is judged by another student at the same level.

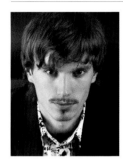

Pencil moustache – PEN-suhl muh-STAHSH – Also known as mouthbrow, this is a thin, narrow, closely clipped moustache that outlines the upper lip. It can be clipped into slight variations to suit facial features.

Penetrating conditioners – PEN-uh-tray-ting kuhn-DISH-uhn-uhz – Products designed to repair and strengthen the physical structure of the hair. The ingredients would normally include quaternary ammonium compounds, proteins (amino acids), humectants (to lock in moisture) and emollients (to soften and smooth the hair).

Percentage strength – puh-SEN-tij STRENGTH – This is how much of the peroxide solution is peroxide, with the rest as water. For example, in 100g of solution with 12% peroxide, there would be 12g of peroxide and 88g of water.

Performance appraisal – puh-FOR-muhnss uh-PRAY-zuhl – This is a method by which the job performance of an employee is evaluated (generally in terms of quality, quantity, cost and time); it is carried out by a manager or supervisor.

Permanent waving – PUR-muh-nuhnt WAYV-ing – A permanent wave, commonly called a perm, involves the use of chemicals to break some of the disulphide bonds in the hair and then reform them in a different position to produce curly hair.

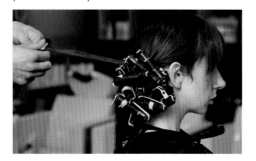

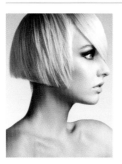

Perimeter – puh-RIM-i-tuh – Length or baseline of the cut.

Perm lotion – PURM LOH-shuhn – A chemical solution that alters the internal structure of the hair, making straight hair curly. The solution works by breaking down the sulphur bonds within the hair shaft.

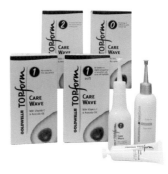

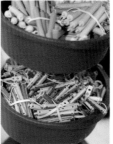

Perm rod – PURM ROD – A tool used to wind the hair around in the perming process.

Perm rubber – PURM RUBB-uh – A rubber band that is used to secure a perm rod.

Perm winding – PURM WIYN-ding – A method of creating curls in the hair with winding techniques, eg brick, directional, spiral, hopscotch. This is used to permanently curl the hair.

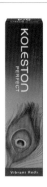

Permanent colour – PURM-uhn-uhnt KUH-luh – Also known as para dyes or oxidation tints, permanent colour can lighten or darken hair, and add tone.

Personal development – PUR-suhn-uhl di-VEL-uhp-muhnt – Taking opportunities to develop your career and learn new skills.

Personal hygiene – PUR-suhn-uhl HIY-jeen – Daily cleansing of the body, face, hands and feet, oral hygiene, and the use of skin and body care products.

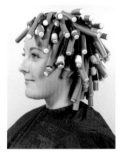

Perming process – PURM-ing PROH-sess – There are three stages in the perming process: softening, moulding and fixing.

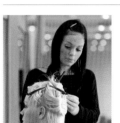

Personal presentation – PUR-suhn-uhl prez-uhn-TAY-shuhn – The image you create with your appearance and personal hygiene.

Peroxide test – puh-ROKS-iyd TEST – A test performed on hair that has had synthetic colour removed. This is used to assess the effectiveness of the process: if the colour removal has been effective, the hair will not change colour, if the hair goes very dark and there is colour change, more synthetic colour will need to be removed.

Personal Protective Equipment (PPE) – PUR-suhn-uhl pruh-TEK-tiv i-KWIP-muhnt -- PEE-PEE-EE – Equipment available for use in the workplace to protect you, your skin and clothes from damage. For example, gloves, apron and uniform.

Peroxometer – puh-roks-OM-uh-tuh – When diluting peroxide, the diluted solution can be checked with a peroxometer.

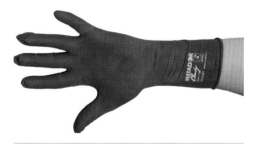

Personal space – PUR-suhn-uhl SPAYSS – The space or 'aura' around a person. Many people feel uncomfortable if this space is invaded, so take care not to get too close, as appropriate to the situation. For example, you will obviously be touching your client's face while giving a facial, but that doesn't mean they'd be comfortable with you doing this in the reception area!

Personal survival budget – PUR-suhn-uhl suh-VIY-vuhl BUJ-it – The amount of money needed to maintain a reasonable and realistic lifestyle.

Personal targets – PUR-suhn-uhl TAH-gits – Individually agreed development goals and targets for each staff member to work towards.

Petrissage – PET-ri-sahzh or pet-ri-SAHZH – A massage movement used during the conditioning process this is used to stimulate the scalp. The massage is a slow, firm, deep kneading movement.

pH balance – pee-AICH BAL-unhss – The normal pH of the hair and skin's surface is 4.5–5.5. Perming can affect this, so pH-balancing products are used after perming to return the hair and skin to 4.5–5.5.

pH paper – pee-AICH PAY-puh – Also known as litmus paper – its main use is to test whether a solution is acidic or alkaline.

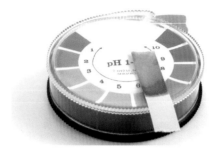

pH scale – pee-AICH SKAYL – A scale that ranges from 1–14. Acid has a pH lower than 7, alkaline has a pH higher than 7, and pH 7 is neutral.

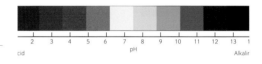

Pharmacist – FAH-muh-sist – A person who is an expert in medicines and their use. They are licensed to prepare and dispense drugs and non-prescription drugs that are safe to be sold over the counter.

Pheomelanin – FEE-oh-MEL-uh-nin – The natural red and yellow pigments that produce warm tones in the hair.

Physical damage – FIZ-ikl DAM-ij – Damage to the hair caused by sun, wind and electrical goods.

Piggyback wind – PIG-ee-bak WIYND – A weaved section of hair is left out while the rest of the section is wound to the roots; then a different size of rod is used to wind the weaved section, placing it to sit on the top.

Pigment – PIG-muhnt – The substance that colours our tissue (hair and skin).

Pin curl weft – PIN KURL weft – A small postiche of curls woven and secured to a hairpin for easy attachment to the head.

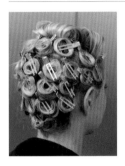

Pin curling – PIN kur-ling – A setting technique used to curl or wave the hair and add volume; a spring clip or pin is used to secure the set.

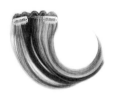

Pin wave – PIN wayv – A small waved postiche woven and secured to a hairpin for easy attachment to the head.

Pityriasis capitis – pit-ee-RY-uh-sis kuh-PIY-tiss – This condition is commonly known as dandruff. The cause is overactive production and shedding of the epidermal cells. This can be identified by small, itchy, dry scales (white or grey).

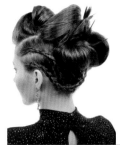

Plaiting and twisting techniques – PLAT-ing uhnd TWIST-ing tek-NEEKS – On scalp plaits, off scalp plaits, and twists.

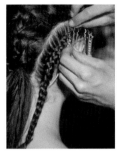

Plaiting technique – PLAT-ing tek-NEEK – A single plait, using three strands of hair, and a fishtail plait, using two strands of hair.

Plan for creating an image – PLAN fuh kree-AY-ting uhn IM-ij – The plan for creating an image will include making a design plan and producing a storyboard or mood board.

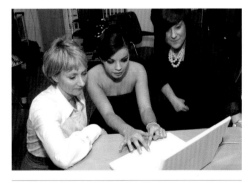

Planning – PLAN-ing – It is crucial that you carry out good planning before a photo shoot, hair show or other event. Poor planning results in poor performance.

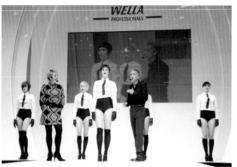

Platysma muscle – pluh-TIZ-muh MUSSL – The platysma is a broad sheet of muscle arising from the chest and shoulders, and rising over the collarbone.

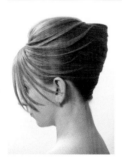

Pleat – PLEET – The pleat is also known as a vertical roll of hair: a long roll usually worn at the back of the head. It is most suitable for long hair but can be achieved with mid-length hair.

Point cutting – POYNT KUT-ing – A method of cutting the ends of the hair to a point.

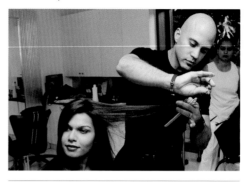

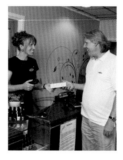

Point of sale (POS) – POYNT uhv SAYL – Usually the location where the credit/debit card transaction is processed, with the customer present. POS is also used as a broad term to describe the location where something is purchased.

Point to root – POYNT tuh ROOT – A method of creating curl movement in the hair by winding the rollers in a traditional way (tip to root).

Policies and procedures – POL-uh-siz uhnd pruh-SEED-yuhz – Employers have these in place to protect you: they cover personal presentation, safe working and what to do in an emergency.

Polite manner – puh-LIYT MAN-uh – It's always crucial to adopt a polite manner when dealing with clients, which includes smiling, and saying 'please' and 'thank you'. Clients are more likely to return to the salon if they have been politely treated.

Polypeptide – pol-ee-PEP-tyd – This is derived from poly (many) and peptos (broken down).

Polypeptide chain – po-lee-PEP-tiyd CHAYN – Formed of many amino acids and peptide bonds, these are held together by permanent and temporary bonds inside the cortex layer of the hair.

Porosity test – por-ROSS-it-ee TEST – A test of the hair's capacity to absorb or resist moisture.

Porous – POR-ruhss – Absorbs liquid.

Portfolio – port-FOH-lee-oh – A collection of your work that could include photographs, sketches, testimonials from satisfied clients and any appearances of your work in magazines.

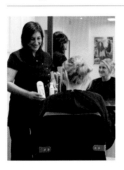

Positive attitude – POZ-it-iv AT-it-yood – Demonstrated with good body language, making eye contact, smiling and tone of voice.

Positive body language – POZ-it-iv BO-dee LANG-gwij – Non-spoken communication such as posture, gesture or facial expression. An example of positive body language is smiling and looking at the person talking to you.

Positive image – POZ-it-iv IM-ij – In order to create a positive image at the reception, you must consider your personal appearance and behaviour, give an efficient reception service, ensure a clean and tidy reception and display area, and meet and greet clients appropriately.

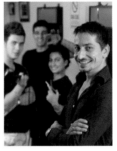

Positive impression – POZ-it-iv im-PRESH-uhn – It is important that the client is impressed with your professional attitude and believes that you have presented a good image of yourself and your salon. Satisfied clients are more likely to return to the salon, so it's really important to give a positive impression.

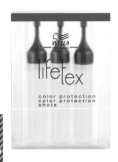

Post-colouring treatment
– POHST-KUH-luh-ring TREET-muhnt – A conditioner that helps to prevent the colour from fading; the treatment closes the cuticles, restores the hair to its natural pH balance and stops oxidation.

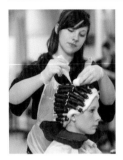

Post-damping
– POHST-DAM-ping – A method of applying perm lotion – the hair is fully wound before the perm lotion is applied.

Post-perm conditioner – POHST-purm kuhn-DISH-uhn-uh – A product used after the perm to close the cuticle, lock in moisture and bring the hair back to the correct pH of 4.5–5.5.

Post-perm treatment – POHST-purm TREET-muhnt – An anti-oxidant surface conditioner used after perming to smooth the cuticle scales, stop creeping oxidation and restore the hair back to its natural pH balance.

Post-treatment – POHST-TREET-muhnt – Will bring the hair back to its normal pH level and replace lost moisture.

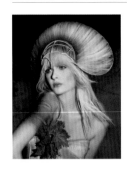

Postiche –
poss-TEESH – A hairpiece added to the hairstyle for creative effects and ornamentation.

Posture – POSS-chuh – The way we stand and hold ourselves. It is important to stand correctly while working so that you don't get tired or injure yourself. It is recommended that you stand with your feet hip-width apart and keep your back straight – try not to bend or stretch too much.

Potassium hydroxide – puh-TASS-ee-uhm hiy-DROKS-iyd – A chemical occasionally used in hair relaxers.

Potentially infectious condition – puh-TEN-shuh-lee in-FEK-shuhss kuhn-DISH-uhn – A condition that may cause visible signs of swelling, or redness on the skin, and may spread, eg bacteria, viruses or fungi.

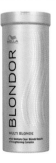

Powder bleach
– POW-duh BLEECH – There are a variety of powder bleaches to choose from, eg blue powder, white powder and powder granules.

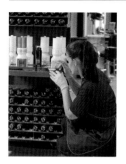

PPE – PEE-PEE-EE – Personal Protective Equipment refers to equipment available for use in the workplace to protect you from harm and damage, eg gloves and an apron are used in hairdressing salons.

Pre-blended oils – PREE-BLEN-did OYLZ – Pre-mixed oils added to the scalp during the massage technique.

Pre-colouring treatment – PREE-KUH-luh-ring TREET-muhnt – A product applied to the hair before a colour service to even out the porosity of the hair.

Pre-damping – PREE-DAM-ping – A method of applying perm lotion to the hair before winding perm rods into the hair. Normally used on long hair to make sure you get even penetration of the perm lotion.

Pre-disposition test – pree-diss-puh-ZISH-uhn TEST – Also known as a skin test, this is used to check if a client is allergic to a colour product.

Pre-lighten – PREE-LIY-tuhn – A lightening product used when the required amount of lift cannot be achieved using permanent high lift colour.

Pre-perm conditioner – PREE-PURM kuhn-DISH-uh-nuh – A conditioner that evens out the porosity of the hair prior to perming.

Pre-perm shampoo – PREE-PURM sham-POO – A shampoo designed to be used before a perm, containing no conditioning additives that may form a barrier against the perm.

Pre-perm treatment – PREE-PURM TREET-muhnt – A product applied to the hair prior to a chemical service to even out the porosity along the hair shaft.

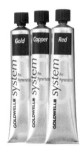

Pre-pigmentation – PREE-pig-men-TAY-shuhn – Reintroduction of gold, copper or red tones in the hair (depending on existing base and target colour), prior to application of the new colour.

Pre-softening – PREE-SOF-uh-ning – A method of applying a weak solution of liquid hydrogen peroxide to resistant hair. This will lift and open the cuticles, allowing the colouring products to penetrate the hair.

Pre-treatment – PREE-TREET-muhn – Coating the cuticle with a polymer film, which acts as a buffer to slow down the chemical product.

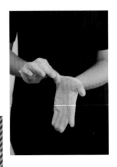

Precautions – pri-KOR-shuhnz – To keep yourself safe, following all health and safety guidelines.

Precision cut – pri-SIZH-uhn KUT – A cut that uses strong, accurate, clearly defined lines, such as a geometric cut.

Prepare the work area – pri-PAIR dhuh WURK AIR-ee-uh – Arranging products, tools and equipment ready for the service to follow.

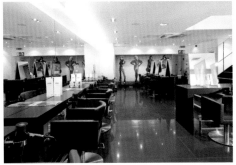

Presentation methods – prez-uhn-TAY-shuhn METH-uhdz – Methods used to explain concepts and ideas, such as a short talk using Powerpoint slides.

Presentation/sales presentation – prez-uhn-TAY-shuhn/SAYLZ prez-uhn-TAY-shuhn – The process of explaining the product or service to the client, ideally including the product's features, advantages and benefits.

Presenting a created image – pri-ZEN-ting uh kree-AY-tid IM-ij – You can present an image as part of a show, a competition, a presentation or a photographic shoot.

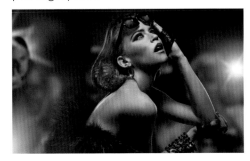

Pressing – PRESS-ing – A method of straightening the hair with heated equipment, for example a pressing comb or flat irons.

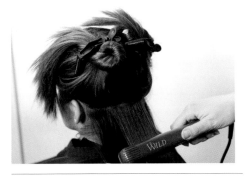

Pressing comb – PRESS-ing KOHM – A heated comb used to stretch and comb the hair straight.

Prices Act – PRIY-siz akt – The price of products must be displayed so that the client is not given the wrong or false information on the product.

Prickle cells – PRIKL SELZ – A cell in the germinal layer of the skin.

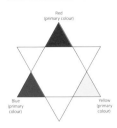

Red
(primary colour)

Blue
(primary colour)

Yellow
(primary colour)

Primary colours – PRIY-muh-ree KUH-luhz – Red, yellow and blue are the three colour pigments that cannot be made up from other colours. When mixing any two of these colours, secondary colours are produced, for example red plus yellow equals orange.

Processing time – PROH-sess-ing TIYM – The development time for a service.

Product build-up – PROD-uhkt BILD-up – When the hair has had excessive products applied, even though the hair is shampooed, the products still remain.

Productivity – prod-uhk-TIV-it-ee – This means the amount of work that you are getting done. If you work effectively, you will achieve high productivity.

Products – PROD-uhkts – Substances we use on our hair every day, eg shampoo, conditioner, styling gel and hairspray.

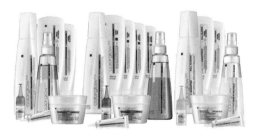

Professional advice – pruh-FESH-uh-nuhl uhd-VYSS – Giving advice to a person based on your skills, knowledge and professional experiences.

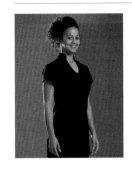

Professional image – pruh-FESH-uh-nuhl IM-ij – Presenting yourself well in the salon, including following the rules of the dress code and using positive body language.

Professional indemnity insurance – pruh-FESH-uh-nuhl in-DEM-nit-ee in-SHOR-ruhnss – This will cover the salon against damages: for example, a customer might claim damages if their scalp is burned by incorrectly mixed chemicals.

Profit and loss – PROF-it uhnd LOSS – A financial statement that summarises the financial transactions for a business over a period in time.

Prominent and protruding – PROM-in-uhnt uhnd pruh-TROO-ding – Sticking out.

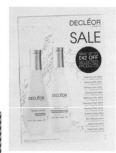

Promotions
– pruh-MOH-shuhnz – Ways of informing the client about products or services to increase interest and, if relevant, sales.

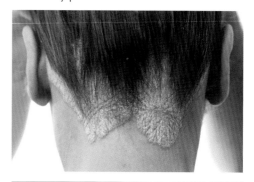

Protective equipment for clients
– pruh-TEK-tiv i-KWIP-muhnt fuh KLIY-uhnts – Gown, towels, waterproof cape, cotton wool and barrier cream.

Protein conditioners –
PROH-teen kuhn-DISH-uh-nuhz – Hair restructurants are protein conditioners, containing protein hydrolysates.

Proteins – PROH-teenz – The essential constituents of living beings; the main protein in the hair is called keratin.

Protofibrils – PROH-toh-FIY-brilz –
In a single strand of hair, three alpha helices are twisted together to form a protofibril – these fibres are found in the cortex and determine the elasticity, strength and thickness of the hair.

Provision and use of work equipment regulations – pruh-VIZH-uhn uhnd YOOSS uhv WURK i-KWIP-mhnt reg-yuh-LAY-shuhnz –
Employers must ensure that all who use the equipment have been adequately trained. You must ensure that you are competent when using tools and equipment in the salon.

Psoriasis – suh-RIY-uh-siss – An inflamed abnormal thickening of the skin, which can be seen as red, itchy and scaly patches.

Public Liability Insurance – PUB-lik liy-uh-BIL-it-ee in-SHOR-ruhnss – This insurance covers slips, falls and any other accidents which cause an injury to a member of the public or customer, or which damage their property.

Pull burn – PUUL BURN – When a perm rod has been wound too tight, it pulls the neck of the follicle open and allows the perm solution to enter the follicle opening. This may become infected, causing folliculitis.

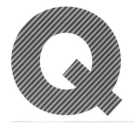

Pull test – PUUL TEST – A test that will help you to evaluate excessive hair loss. Separate a handful of hair and gently pull at the roots – if more than 12 hairs are lost this may be an indication of abnormal hair loss.

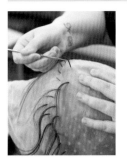

Pull through highlights and lowlights – PUUL THROO HIY-liyts uhnd LOH-liyts – Colouring techniques that colour parts of the hair using a variety of methods, including cap, spatulas, colour cups and strips.

Purchaser – PUR-chiss-uh – Someone who buys a product.

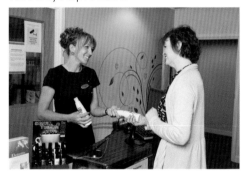

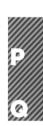

Quality management – KWOL-it-ee MAN-ij-muhnt – The implementation of effective systems and procedures relating to tasks carried out each day in the salon.

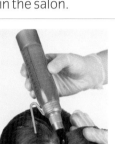

Quasi-permanent colour – KWAH-zee-PUR-muh-nuhnt KUH-luh – Colour that lasts almost as long as a permanent one. It should be treated as permanent colour in terms of testing and future services.

Questioning – KWES-chuh-ning – Open questions are used when you need to gain information and need to keep a conversation going, eg who, what, when, how. Closed questions are used when you wish to summarise and move on; they will be answered by yes or no.

Questionnaire

Questionnaire – kwess-chuh-NAIR – A method of collecting feedback from clients to be used for evaluation purposes.

Quiff – KWIF – Where the hair is cut longer at the front fringe area, so the hair can be styled back off the face.

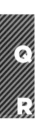

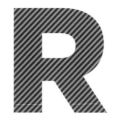

Race Relations Act – RAYSS ri-LAY-shuhnz akt – Protects people from discrimination on the grounds of colour, race, nationality or ethnic origins.

Rake – RAYK – A large wide-toothed comb.

Rapport – rap-OR – Working in harmony and agreement.

Razor – RAY-zuh – A tool used to remove bulk or to thin out the ends. They are especially handy for creating a textured look.

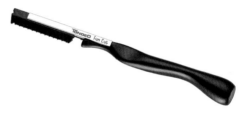

Rebookings – ree-BUUK-ingz – Clients who remain loyal to the salon but are happy to see any hairdresser.

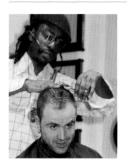

Receding hairline – ri-SEE-ding HAIR-liyn – Hair receding from the lateral sides of the forehead.

Reception – ri-SEP-shuhn – This is the area where clients book and make payments for services.

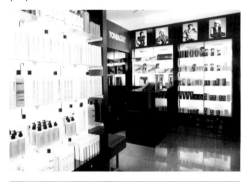

Reception stationery – ri-SEP-shuhn STAY-shun-uh-ree – Writing materials such as pencils, rubbers, message pads and appointment cards.

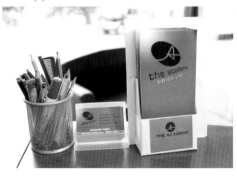

Receptionist – ri-SEP-shuhn-ist – In a salon or spa, this person greets clients and also makes the appointments for the services and treatments being carried out. They may also be responsible for answering any enquiries made by clients.

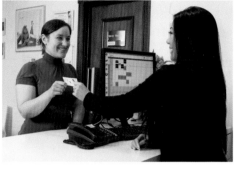

Reclining chair – ri-KLIY-ning CHAIR – A chair that has a varied backwards and forwards movement, mainly used in hairdressing salons at the backwash area.

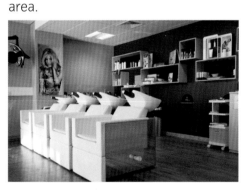

Record card – REK-ord KAHD – A log of all the services that have taken place on the client's hair. The log will include mixing ratios, strengths of products used, time limits, shampoo, conditioners, styling products and chemical services.

Reducing agent – ruh-DYOO-sing AY-juhnt – A product that adds hydrogen to the hair; this can be found in perm lotion and colour reducers.

Reduction – ruh-DUK-shuhn – The addition of hydrogen to the hair. The chemical process of softening the hair to shape it around the perm rod – the first stage of perming.

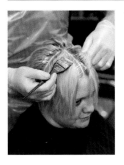

Referral – ri-FUR-ruhl – When a client is advised to seek further advice on something from a person more knowledgeable in the subject; for example, if a client had visible signs of head lice, you would refer them to a pharmacist.

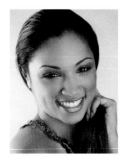

Regrowth application – REE-GROHTH ap-li-KAY-shuhn – Applying colour to the roots where colour has grown out.

Regulations – reg-yuh-LAY-shuhnz – If Parliament passes an Act, for example the Health and Safety at Work Act, we have to know which rules to follow. These rules are called regulations.

Regulatory Reform (Fire Safety) Order 2005 – REG-yuh-la-TOR-ree reh-FORM (FIY-uh SAYF-tee) OR-duh TOO-OH-OH-FIYV – Employers must ensure that a fire risk assessment is carried out for the workplace by a competent person and that suitable arrangements are in place for fire detection, fire fighting, employee training and emergency evacuation. All equipment must be regularly maintained and evacuation routes must be kept clear at all times.

Relaxing – ruh-LAKS-ing – A chemical treatment where the natural curl or movement from a client's hair is removed or reduced. This may be temporary or permanent.

Relevant person – REL-uh-vuhnt PUR-suhn – The person who you would report to or seek advice from.

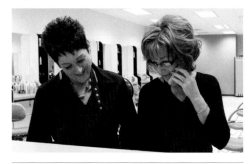

Removal of colouring products – ri-MOO-vuhl uhv KUH-luh-ring PROD-uhkts – After full development time, add water to the tint on the head and emulsify, lifting the tint from the scalp, then rinse, shampoo and condition.

Remy hair – RAY-mee HAIR – Hair that has been cut from the head and the cuticles are all lying in the same direction.

Repetitive Strain Injury (RSI) –
ri-PET-uh-tiv STRAYN IN-juh-ree --
AH ESS IY – Injury resulting from doing
one type of action too much. The wrist
and fingers are especially prone to RSI.

**Reporting of Injuries, Diseases
and Dangerous Occurrences
Regulations (RIDDOR)** – ri-POR-ting
uhv IN-juh-riz diz-EE-ziz unhd DAYN-juh-
ruhss uh-KURR-uhn-siz reg-yuh-LAY-
shuhnz -- RID-or – If you or your client
suffer from personal injury at work then
it must be reported in the salon accident
book. This is to inform the employer and
so that serious injury may be reported
to the local enforcement officer.

Resale Price Act – REE-sayl PRYS
akt – This act prevents manufacturers
from imposing a specified retail price
for goods. It is unlawful for a supplier
to impose a minimum retail price by
withholding supplies of the goods
or discriminating in any other way.
Many companies do however have
a recommended retail price which
they suggest their customers use.

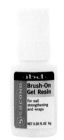

Resin – RE-zin –
An adhesive used
to bond some
extensions on to
the natural hair.

Resistant hair – ruh-ZISS-tuhnt HAIR –
Hair that is difficult to alter chemically.

Resources – ruh-ZOR-siz – All the
things in a salon that make the service
possible, eg tools, equipment,
products, gowns, towels, etc.

Respiratory problems – ruh-SPI-ruh-
tree PROB-luhmz – Breathing problems.

Responsibilities – ruh-spon-suh-
BIL-it-eez – The duties that a person
within a particular job role is expected
to perform.

Responsible person – ruh-SPON-sibl
PUR-suhn – Someone who has control,
or a degree of control, over the work
environment.

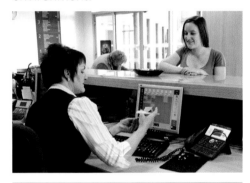

Restore depth and tone – ri-STOR
DEPTH uhnd TOHN – Recolouring the
hair by adding depth and brightness.

Restructurant – ree-STRUK-chuh-ruhnt – Restructurants are designed to penetrate the cortex in order to strengthen and repair the very inner part of the hair follicle.

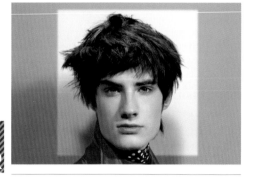

Restyle – REE-STYL – To completely change the style for the client; to produce a new look.

Retail displays
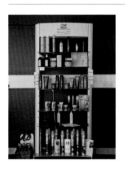
– REE-tayl diss-PLAYZ – A colourful, clean, tidy and eye-catching display of all the products and tools that are available for sale to the clients.

Return clients – ruh-TURN KLIY-uhnts – Clients that have returned to the same stylist and remain loyal to them.

Reverse graduation – ri-VURSS grad-yoo-AY-shuhn – Once the initial guideline has been cut, each subsequent section is cut slightly longer.

Reverse pin curling – ri-VURSS PIN KUR-ling – When the first row is placed in one direction (curling to the left), and when you progress onto the next section, placing the pin curls in the opposite direction (curling to the right).

Ringworm – RING-wurm – A highly infectious fungal skin infection that should not be treated in the salon, starting with grey whitish skin surrounded by small, round red spots, growing into larger spots with a raised scaly border. The hair often falls out, creating bald patches. This is also known as tinea capitis.

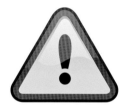

Risk – RISK – The likelihood of harm: if a wire is trailing across a passageway there is a high risk of someone tripping over it, but if it lies along a wall out of the way, the risk is far smaller.

Risk assessment – RISK uh-SESS-muhnt – This is a careful examination of what could cause harm to people in a particular location, such as a photo shoot set. You should do this so you can weigh up whether you have taken enough precautions or should do more to prevent harm.

Role – ROHL – The actions and activities expected of a person within a particular job.

Rollering – ROH-luh-ring – Velcro rollers or those secured with pins are amongst the many types of rollers available. They are all used to create volume, curl and/or movement in the hair.

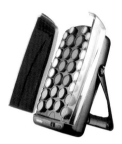

Rollers – ROH-luhz – There are many varieties of rollers, such as heated rollers, spiral rollers, conventional setting rollers, foam rollers, velcro rollers and bendies.

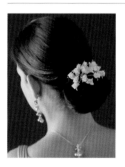

Rolls – ROHLZ – A chignon is a good example of a roll in the nape of the neck. Rolls can be placed anywhere on the head depending on the effect that is to be achieved.

Root drag – ROOT drag – The hair is lifted away from the head at an angle less or greater than 90° from the root area.

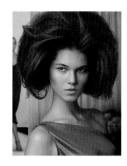

Root lift – ROOT lift – Lifting the hair upwards and away from the root area to give body and height to the style.

Root perm – ROOT purm – A technique of winding the root area of the hair only around the perm rod to give root lift only.

Root to point – ROOT tuh POYNT – A method of creating curl or movement in hair by winding on spiral rollers or tongs, starting at the hair from the root and finishing at the ends. Pin curls can also be achieved with this method.

Rotary – ROH-turr-ee – A firm, circular massage movement, using the pads of the fingers on the scalp during the shampooing process. Used to cleanse the hair.

Rounded neckline – ROWN-did NEK-liyn – A neckline where the corners have been cut off; the back of the hairline is cut into the shape of a horseshoe.

R

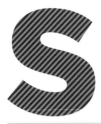

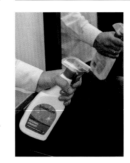

Safe working practices – SAYF WUR-king PRAK-tiss-iz – It is very important to work safely and hygienically at all times when working in the salon.

Sabouraud-Rousseau test – SAB-oo-roh ROO-soh TEST – Also known as a skin test, this is used to check if a client is allergic to a colour product.

Safe and hygienic working practices – SAYF uhnd hiy-JEE-nik WUR-king PRAK-tiss-iz – To work safely and hygienically in the salon, you must use the PPE provided, follow COSHH, use appropriate methods of sterilisation, and follow the relevant health and safety legislation.

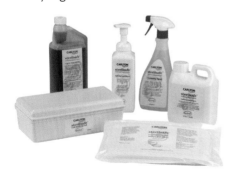

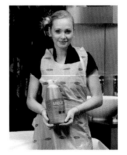

Safety considerations – SAYF-tee kuhn-sid-uh-RAY-shuhnz – You need to ensure that you carry out the right preparation, follow COSHH, use safe working methods, use or wear your provided PPE and follow the manufacturer's instructions when using products or equipment.

Safe working methods – SAYF WUR-king METH-uhdz – Working in a way that will not increase the risk of someone in your workplace being injured.

Safety Data Sheet – SAYF-tee DAY-tuh SHEET – Provides information on chemical products that helps users of those chemicals to make a risk assessment. It describes the hazards the chemical presents and gives information on handling, storage and emergency measures in case of an accident.

Sale and Supply of Goods Act – SAYL uhnd suh-PLY uhv GUUDZ akt – As a seller, you must ensure that the goods you sell are of satisfactory quality, fit for purpose and do anything you claim they can do.

Sale of Goods Act – SAYL uhv GUUDZ akt – Retail products must be of good quality, do what they claim to do, and fit their description.

Sales forecast – SAYLZ FOR-kahst – Prediction of the future sales of a particular product, including treatments over a specific period of time based on past performance of the product, inflation rates, unemployment, consumer spending patterns, market trends and interest rates.

Sales techniques – SALYZ tek-NEEKS – Ways in which you will help the client to decide the product or service that will suit their needs.

Salon junior – SAL-o(ng) or suh-LO(ng) JOO-nee-uh – A person who is employed to help the senior members of staff in a salon or spa. Their duties will include shampooing the hair or preparing the work area for a beauty treatment.

Salon manager – SAL-o(ng) or suh-LO(ng) MAN-i-juh – This person is in charge of the day-to-day running of the salon, for example making decisions on staff responsibilities and recruitment of employees.

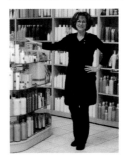

Salon owner – SAL-o(ng) or suh-LO(ng) OH-nuh – A person who owns a salon business and makes important decisions regarding the overall running of the salon.

Salon policy – SAL-o(ng) or suh-LO(ng) POL-i-see – The procedures and requirements for salon processes and systems, for example staff grievances or client refunds.

Salon procedures – SAL-o(ng) or suh-LO(ng) pruh-SEED-yuhz – The rules and systems that your salon has in place, of which your supervisor will inform you.

Salon requirements – SAL-o(ng) or suh-LO(ng) ruh-KWIY-uh-muhnts – The rules and regulations issued by the salon manager.

Salon services – SAL-o(ng) or suh-LO(ng) SUR-viss-iz – The services that are offered by the salon.

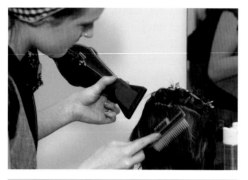

Salon standards – SAL-o(ng) or suh-LO(ng) STAN-duhdz – Your manager will show you how he/she expects you to dress and behave. There may be a salon dress code or uniform and a salon code of conduct, which states how you should look and behave.

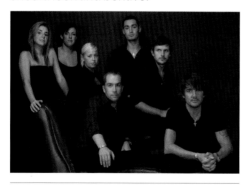

Salt bonds – SOLT bondz – Temporary bonds in the hair structure.

Sanitisation – san-it-iy-ZAY-shuhn – The equipment you use should be in a hygienic condition before use, which means sanitising and sterilising it. Methods of doing this include using a UV cabinet.

Sanitise – SAN-i-tiyz – To make hygienic and clean by destroying most micro-organisms.

Scabies – SKAY-beez – This condition is caused by a reaction to an itch mite. The tiny animal parasite (sarcoptes scabiei) burrows through the skin and lays its eggs. The areas affected become extremely itchy, especially at night. There are reddish spots and burrows (greyish lines) under the skin. Refer sufferers to a doctor.

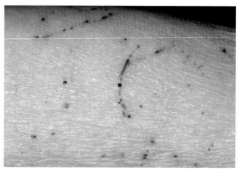

Scalp – SKALP – The head area, surrounded by the face and the neck.

Scalp irritation – SKALP irr-i-TAY-shuhn – The scalp has reacted to a product or service, showing signs of redness, itchiness and inflammation.

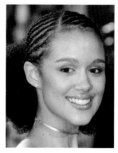

Scalp plait – SKALP PLAT – There are three types of plait that sit on their own base: the French plait, canerows and cornrows.

Scalp treatment – SKALP TREET-muhnt – Products applied to the scalp to treat a specific condition, eg a greasy scalp.

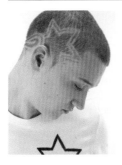

Scalpting – SKALP-ting – The cutting of shapes into the hair close to the scalp.

Scar tissue – SKAH TISH-yoo – Dense fibrous connective tissue that forms over and/or around a healed wound or cut.

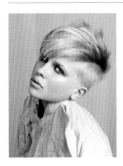

Scissor over comb – SIZ-uh OH-vuh KOHM – A technique used to cut the hair very short, following the natural contours of the head. The hair is lifted and held in the comb by combing the hair in an upward motion, and the hair that protrudes through the comb is cut, holding the scissors above the comb.

Scrunch dry – SKRUNCH DRIY – Finger drying the hair, creating lift, volume and curl with the aid of a diffuser.

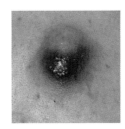

Sebaceous cyst – si-BAY-shuhss SIST – A lump of fibrous tissues and fluids. The most common sites for sebaceous cysts are the scalp, back and face.

Sebaceous glands – si-BAY-shuss GLANDZ – Glands in the skin that secrete oil.

Seborrhoea – seb-uh-REE-uh – Overactive sebaceous glands of the scalp, leading the hair and scalp to become excessively greasy.

Seborrhoeic dermatitis – seb-uh-REE-ik dur-muh-TIY-tiss – Inflammation of the skin (grease glands) where a rash forms in areas such as the side of the nose, forehead and scalp.

Sebum – SEE-buhm – An oily, waxy substance secreted by the sebaceous glands.

Secondary colours – SEK-uhn-dree KUH-luhz – Violet, green and orange are each made up from two primary colours. Red and blue make violet.

Secondary tone – SEK-uhn-dree TOHN – This is the second number when looking at hair tone. So, for hair tone /34, the 3 is the primary tone and the 4 is the secondary tone.

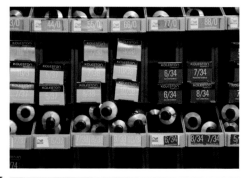

Section marks – SEK-shuhn mahks – Marks in the hair that have been dried in place by a setting roller.

Sectioning – SEK-shuhn-ing – This is the process of making a clean parting in the hair; sectioning the hair allows you to work in a controlled manner.

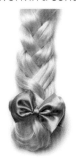

Securing the hair – si-KYOO-uh-ring dhuh HAIR – Ensuring that the plait stays in place by using bands, ribbons or clips.

Seepage – SEEP-ij – The product from the foil package has seeped out, colouring the hair that was outside of the package.

Self-assessment – self-uh-SESS-muhnt – Students making judgments about their own work.

Self-employed – SELF-im-PLOYD – Working for yourself and no longer working for somebody else, eg freelance hairdresser.

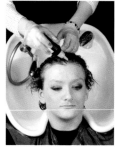

Semi-permanent – SEM-ee-PUR-muh-nuhnt – Colour that lasts for six to eight washes. Ideal for clients who would like to colour their hair but are unsure about maintaining permanent colour.

Senegalese twist – sen-uh-guh-LEEZ TWIST – A rope effect plait, achieved with two strands of hair twisted in the same direction.

Sensitised hair – SENS-it-iyzd HAIR – Hair that is delicate because chemical services have damaged its internal structure.

Sensitivity test – SEN-sit-iv-it-ee TEST – sometimes referred to as a skin patch test, this is a test carried out 24 hours before the treatment to see if the client is allergic to certain products, eg tinting products and perming products.

Serrated scissors – suh-RAY-tid SIZ-uhz – Also known as thinning scissors, used to thin the hair.

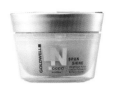

Serum – SEER-uhm – A product used to add shine and moisture to the hair.

Service plan – SUR-viss PLAN – A record of services performed, the outcomes and recommendations given.

Services – SUR-viss-iz – The different types of hairdressing offered to clients in salons, such as cutting or colouring.

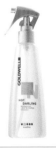

Setting lotion – SET-ing LOH-shuhn – A product used to lengthen the life of the set; it is applied prior to a set.

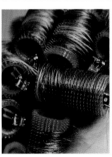

Setting rollers – SET-ing ROH-luhz – A tool that is used to create curls, volume or hair direction.

Sewn-in extensions – SOHN-IN iks-TEN-shuhnz – In the underneath layer of your hair, this is the sewing of the extensions to a cornrow braid across your scalp. This is an effective method, as little damage is done to natural hair; they are securely held onto the scalp and can be easily removed by cutting the thread.

Sex Discrimination Act – SEKS dis-krim-i-NAY-shuhn akt – Protects anyone against discrimination based on their sexuality.

Shade chart – SHAYD CHAHT – Also known as an international colour chart – it shows depth of colour (2–10) and tone of colour (natural, gold, red, copper, brunette, ash).

Shades – SHAYDZ – Different tones in the hair, eg red, copper, gold and brunette.

Shampoo – sham-POO – A product that cleans the hair and scalp.

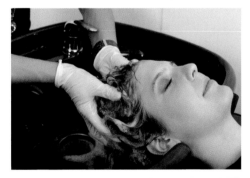

Sharps

Sharps – SHAHPS – A term used by the Health and Safety Executive to describe sharp objects, for example scissors, razors and razor blades, that may have by-laws covering their disposal.

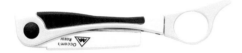

Shine spray – SHIYN spray – A finishing product applied to the hair to enhance the sheen.

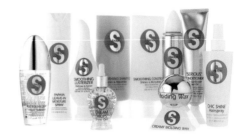

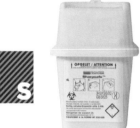

Sharps box
– SHAHPS boks – The sharps box is where all used 'sharps' (ie blades) must be disposed of.

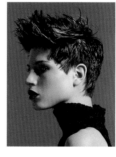

Shingles –
SHING-guhlz – Also known as herpes zoster, this virus also causes chickenpox and can be identified by painful skin blisters on the body.

Shaving brushes – SHAY-ving BRUSH-iz – Often made of badger hair and used to lather and apply shaving products.

Shaving creams – SHAY-ving KREEMZ – A moisturising product designed to create a thick lather. These must be applied before shaving.

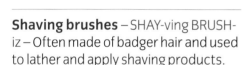

Short graduation
– SHORT grad-yoo-AY-shuhn – The inner layers of the hair lengths are longer than the outline shape.

Shaving oils – SHAY-ving OYLZ – Oils specially designed for application before shaving. They lubricate and moisturise the face.

Shimmering – SHIM-uh-ring – This is a method of colouring the ends/tips of the hair.

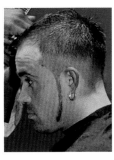

Sideburns – SIYD-burnz – Sideburns are the areas of facial hair that grow down the sides of the face, in front of the ears. They can be worn alone or can connect the hair of the scalp with the rest of the facial hair.

Skin staining – SKIN stay-ning – The tint applied to the hair has stained the skin. This is the result of a poor application.

Skin structure – SKIN STRUK-chuh – The skin is the largest organ of the body. The skin has two main layers – the epidermis and dermis – and below these is a layer of subcutaneous fat.

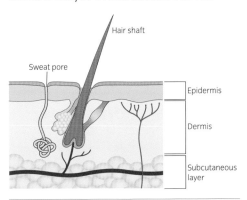

Hair shaft

Sweat pore

Epidermis

Dermis

Subcutaneous layer

Skin tensioning – SKIN TEN-shuhn-ing – The tension applied to the skin when performing facial shaving services.

Skin test – SKIN TEST – Also known as a patch test and hypersensitivity test. This is a test to check to see if the client is allergic to the product used.

Slicing – SLIY-sing – A technique used to select slices of hair to be coloured.

Small Firms Enterprise Development Initiative – SMORL FURMZ EN-tuh-priyz duh-VEL-uhp-muhnt in-ISH-uh-tiv – The leading organisation for small firms' development and support.

SMART objectives – SMAHT uhb-JEK-tivz – This stands for: Specific, Measurable, Achievable, Realistic, Timebound. This describes how objectives should be written and planned.

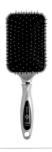

Smoothing – SMOODH-ing – Using tools and equipment to smooth the hair temporarily.

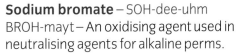

Sodium bromate – SOH-dee-uhm BROH-mayt – An oxidising agent used in neutralising agents for alkaline perms.

Sodium hydroxide-based relaxer (lye) – SOH-dee-uhm hiy-DROK-siyd-baysst ri-LAK-suh -- LIY – This is the stronger of the relaxers, with which you can achieve maximum straightness. There is no mixing of chemicals, there is a varied choice of strengths, and the hair will have more shine.

Soft water – SOFT WOR-tuh – Treated water, without limescale. Soft water may taste salty and may not be suitable for drinking.

Softening – SOF-uh-ning – The process of applying liquid hydrogen peroxide to resistant hair to open the cuticles.

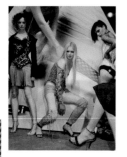

Sources of information (information methods) – SOR-siz uhv in-fuh-MAY-shuhn -- in-fuh-MAY-shuhn METH-uhdz – These include the internet, magazines, photographs, sketches, textbooks, television/DVDs, image libraries and hair/fashion shows.

Soya shampoo – SOY-uh sham-POO – A shampoo used on dry hair, which adds proteins and nutrients to the hair and scalp.

Sparse – SPAHSS – Thinly scattered.

Spatula – SPACH-uh-luh – A tool used to apply colouring products to give a highlighted effect.

Specialist salons – SPESH-uh-list SAH-lo(ng)-z or suh-LO(ng)z – Salons that specialise in certain services, for example African type hairdressing.

Spectrum – SPEK-truhm – The colours in the spectrum are red, orange, yellow, green, blue, indigo and violet.

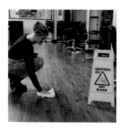

Spillage – SPIL-ij – A product or substance that is dropped or leaked onto the floor.

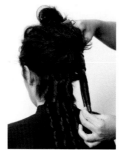

Spiral curling – SPIY-ruhl KUR-ling – A method of winding on rods or tongs from point to root, to achieve a corkscrew effect.

Spiral winding – SPIY-ruhl WIYN-ding – An alternative perm winding technique in which square sections of long hair are wound up a perm rod to form spiral curls. This creates little root lift.

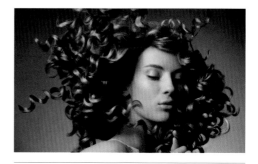

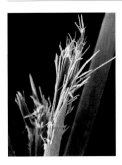

Split ends – SPLIT ENDZ – Also known as fragilitas crinium – when the ends of the hair split into two or three strands. It is normally caused by harsh physical or chemical treatments.

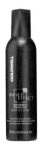

Spray – SPRAY – Helps shorter hairs stay neatly in place when plaiting and twisting. Moisturising sprays can be used on the scalp to prevent it from drying out.

Staff induction – STAHF in-DUK-shuhn – A process to introduce new employees to their jobs and working environment.

Static electricity – STAT-ik uhl-ek-TRISS-it-ee – A build-up of electrical charges in the hair, causing some hairs to have a positive charge, so that they stand up and away from all the other hairs.

Stationery – STAY-shuhn-ree – Resources held at the reception area, eg pens, pencils, notepad, appointment cards, appointment book, price lists and calculator.

Steamer – STEEM-uh – A machine that is used to supply moisture to the hair.

Stem – STEM – The part of a pin curl between the base and the first turn of the circle.

Sterilisation – sterr-i-liy-ZAY-shuhn – The complete destruction of living organisms to prevent cross-infection. All tools should be cleaned before sterilising to remove traces of hair, dirt and dust.

Sterling – STUR-ling – This is the currency used in the UK and is also referred to as the 'Great British Pound' (GBP).

Stock control system – STOK kuhn-TROHL SISS-tuhm – A method of identifying stock levels and tracking stock for the purpose of efficient replenishment; it can be a manual or computerised system.

Stock rotation – STOK roh-TAY-shuhn – Placing new stock at the back of shelves, bringing the old stock forward to use first.

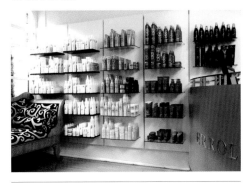

Straightening – STRAYT-ning – Using heated equipment to straighten the hair temporarily.

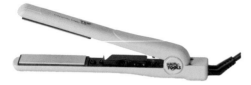

Strand test – STRAND TEST – A test carried out during the colouring service to check the development of a colour. It is used to see if the correct level of lift/depth has been achieved. It is also a test used during a relaxing service to check if the correct level of the straightness has been achieved.

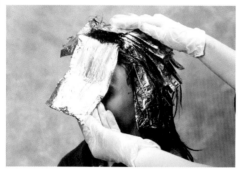

Stratum aculeatum – STRAH-tuhm ak-yoo-lee-AH-tuhm – Also known as stratum spinosum or the skin's prickle cell layer, this is the middle layer of the epidermis.

Stratum corneum – STRAH-tuhm KOR-nee-uhm – Often referred to as the horny layer, the stratum corneum is the top outer layer of the epidermis. It is made up of dead, flattened, keratinised cells that are always being shed.

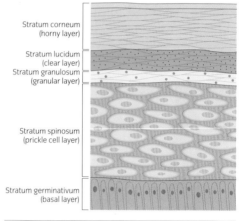

Stratum corneum (horny layer)
Stratum lucidum (clear layer)
Stratum granulosum (granular layer)
Stratum spinosum (prickle cell layer)
Stratum germinativum (basal layer)

Stratum germinativum – STRAH-tuhm jur-min-uh-TIYV-uhm – Often referred to as the basal layer, the stratum germinativum is the bottom layer of the epidermis which attaches to the dermis. It is in this layer that new cells are formed by a process called mitosis.

Stratum granulosum – STRAH-tuhm gran-yoo-LOH-suhm – Often referred to as the granular layer, the stratum granulosum lies beneath the stratum lucidum. It is the layer where keratinisation is completed and the living skin cells are hardened and flattened.

Stratum lucidum – STRAH-tuhm LOO-sid-uhm – Often referred to as the clear layer, the stratum lucidum lies under the stratum corneum and is made up of tightly packed transparent cells. This layer is very thin on the face and thicker on the soles of the feet.

Stratum malpighii – STRAH-tuhm mal-PEE-gee – The major layer of the epidermis, consisting of six to ten layers of keratinocytes.

Stratum spinosum – STRAH-tuhm spin-OH-zuhm or spiyn-OH-zuhm – Also known as stratum aculeatum or the skin's prickle cell layer, this is the middle layer of the epidermis.

Strengths and weaknesses – STRENGTHS uhnd WEEK-niss-iz – Identify these in order to set targets. What are you good at? What do you feel that you need help with?

Stropping – STROP-ing – The aim of stropping is to smooth and shape the razor's edge.

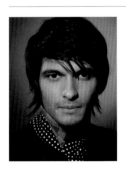

Stubble – STUBL – Very short facial hair, of only one or a few days' growth.

Styling products – STIYL-ing PROD-uhkts – Used to aid in the moulding and drying stage of the set or blow dry, these help protect the hair from heat.

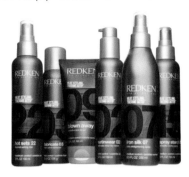

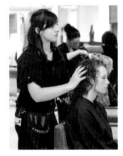

Stylist – STIYL-ist – The person who cuts and styles hair.

Subcutaneous layer – SUB-kyoo-TAYN-ee-uhss LAY-uh – This is found below the dermis and is made up mostly of fat, and helps your body stay warm and absorb shocks.

Sudoriferous gland – soo-duh-RIF-uh-ruhss or syoo-duh-RIF-uh-ruhss GLAND – Sudoriferous glands are glands in the skin that secrete perspiration (produce sweat).

Surface conditioner

Surface conditioner – SUR-fiss kuhn-DISH-uh-nuh – Surface conditioners smooth and coat the cuticles; they do not enter the cortex or strengthen the hair.

Surface conditioning products – SUR-fiss kuhn-DISH-uhn-ing PROD-uhkts – Products designed to add moisture to the hair in order to improve shine and texture. Ingredients would be vegetable and mineral oils, lanolin, fats and waxes, and mild acidic compounds to close the cuticles.

Surface tension – SUR-fiss TEN-shuhn – The skin-like surface layer of a liquid.

Sycosis barbae (barber's itch) – sy-KOH-siss BAH-biy -- BAH-buhz ICH – A bacterial infection of the hairy parts of the face.

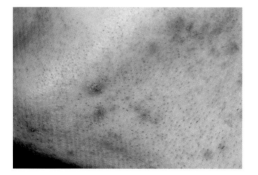

Symmetrical – si-MET-rik-uhl – The same on both sides.

Synthetic dyes – sin-THET-ik DIYZ – A form of permanent colouring also known as para dyes.

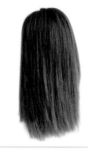

Synthetic hair – sin-THET-ik HAIR – Hair that is not real. This can only be washed in soapy water and must be left to dry naturally.

S

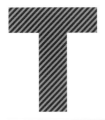

T-liner – TEE-liy-nuh – A clipper with a specially shaped blade used for creating patterns in the hair, for example beards and eyebrows.

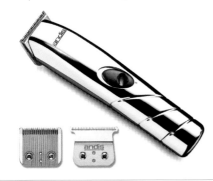

Tangles – TANG-guhlz – Matting or knotting of the hair.

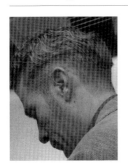

Taper cut – TAY-puh KUT – A taper cut is a short haircut where the sides and back are cut progressively shorter down toward the neck, with even blending throughout.

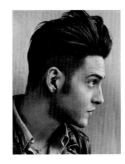

Tapered nape – TAY-puhd nayp – Refers to a gradual decrease in the length of hair at the back of the head, following the natural hairline.

Tapering – TAY-puh-ring – Cutting a fine line into the head shape, for example, when blending layers from the fringe to a longer length at the front of the haircut.

Tapotement – tuh-POHT-muhnt – A gentle tapping of the skin with the pads of the fingertips.

Target – TAH-git – A task to complete – usually within a set timescale – to achieve a particular result. For example, you may be required to sell a number of services or products to meet your salon's sales targets or your own personal goal.

Target group – TAH-git GROOP – The clientele you are trying to attract into the salon; for example, a promotional activity to increase barbering services would be aimed at male clients.

Target setting – TAH-git SET-ing – You and your manager will spend some time discussing your training needs, which will be split into specific, measurable and achievable sections. Your achievement of these targets will be used to measure your progress.

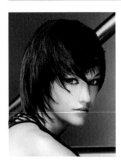

Target shade – TAH-git SHAYD – The colour chosen by the client that the stylist is trying to achieve.

Tea tree oil shampoo – TEE TREE OYL sham-POO – A shampoo that acts like an antiseptic, used to treat some scalp conditions.

Team – TEEM – A group of people who work together.

Team work – TEEM wurk – People working together effectively to achieve a particular aim.

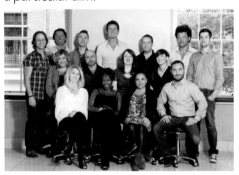

Teasing – TEEZ-ing – After the final look has been achieved, teasing is the replacing of small areas of hair into a new position.

Techniques – tek-NEEKS – These are the different methods used to create the finished image, for example pin curling, finger waving, twisting, knotting, plaiting, weaving and added hair.

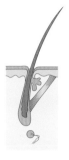

Telogen – TEE-loh-jen or TEL-oh-jen – The resting stage of the hair growth cycle, which can last for 3–4 months.

Temperature – TEM-pruh-chuh – The temperature of a salon will affect chemical services; in a hot salon, the development time of chemical services will be speeded up. The cooler the salon, the slower the development time.

Temporal bones – TEM-puh-ruhl BOHNZ – Situated at the sides and base of the skull, they support the part of the face known as the temple.

Temporalis muscle – tem-puh-RAY-liss or tem-puh-RA-liss MUSSL – A large, thin, curve-shaped muscle positioned in the side of the skull above and in front of the ear.

Temporary products – TEMP-puh-ruh-ree PROD-uhkts – These products will last approximately one shampoo and will add tone, darken natural hair or give a fashion effect.

Tensile strength test – TEN-siyl STRENGTH TEST – Also known as an elasticity test. This is a test to check the strength of the internal structure of the hair.

Tension – TEN-shuhn – How tightly the hair is pulled. Be careful not to pull too much when removing extensions, as damage may occur that could result in hair breakage or even traction alopecia.

Terminal hair – TUR-min-uhl HAIR – The hair on our heads, underarms and genital areas of the body.

Test curl – TEST KURL – A test that is performed during the perming process to check the development of the perm.

Test cutting – TEST KUT-ing – Removing a few strands of hair for processing in order to check the likely results of the selected product.

Texture – TEKS-chuh – The texture of the hair can be assessed as fine, medium or coarse.

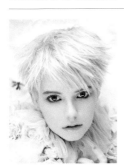

Texturising – TEKS-chuh-riy-zing – Removing small or large amounts of hair to add definition, shape and movement to the style. Scissors or a razor can be used for this.

The Consumer Safety Act – dhuh kuhn-SYOO-muh SAYF-tee akt – This act lays down legal safety standards to minimise the risk to the consumer from potentially harmful or dangerous products.

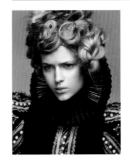

Theme – THEEM – A set subject area; for instance, hair up, fantasy or images reflecting an era, like the seventies or eighties.

Thermal styling – THUR-muhl STIYL-ing – A method of moulding the hair into shapes with heated equipment, for example curling tongs mould the hair into a curl.

Thinning – THIN-ing – Reducing hair bulk without reducing the overall hair length – this can be achieved with scissors or a razor.

Thioglycollate – THIY-oh GLIY-koh-layt – A chemical used in perming and relaxing. The chemicals swell the hair shaft and break down the disulphide bonds in the hair.

Time management – TIYM MAN-ij-muhnt – Organising your time well so that you are as efficient as possible. This can include planning ahead and prioritising your tasks.

Timebound – TIYM-bownd – An activity or objective that has set dates for tasks to be completed or started by.

Tinea capitis – TIN-ee-uh kuh-PIY-tiss – This is commonly known as ringworm of the head. The cause is a fungal infection of the hair and skin. It can be identified by circular grey or white skin, surrounded by red, active rings. The skin looks dull and rough. The condition should be referred to a doctor.

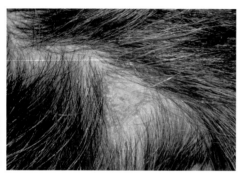

Tinea pedis – TIN-ee-uh PED-iss – This is commonly known as athlete's foot. The cause is a fungus that attacks the skin and can be identified by soft, sore skin, irritation, bleeding and a bad odour. The condition should be referred to a doctor.

Tone – TOHN – The client's hair colour, for example gold, copper or red.

Toner – TOH-nuh – A colour applied to the hair after the lightening process.

Tonging – TONG-ing – A method of curling the hair with heated styling equipment in the shape of a barrel.

Tools – TOOLZ – Combs, brushes, etc used to carry out the hairdressing service.

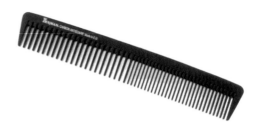

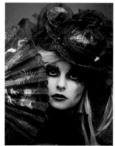

Total look – TOH-tuhl LUUK – In the hair and beauty industry this includes hair, make-up and clothes.

Total price – TOH-tuhl PRYS – When a client buys two or more products or services, add the separate prices together to get the total price.

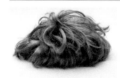

Toupee – TOO-pay – A partial hairpiece, providing hair replacement only over a defined area.

Traction alopecia – TRAK-suhn al-uh-PEE-shuh – Hair thinning or loss due to excessive tension on the hair follicle.

Trades Description Act – TRAYDZ di-SKRIP-shuhn akt – The law stating that products should not falsely or misleadingly describe quality, fitness, price or purpose, by advertisements, displays or description.

Trapezius muscle – truh-PEE-zee-uhss MUSSL – A large muscle that covers the neck, shoulders and back.

Treatment – TREET-muhnt – A process to improve condition – in this instance we mean a penetrating conditioner that improves the cortex condition. It could also be a scalp treatment that remedies a scalp disorder.

Treatment shampoo – TREET-muhnt sham-POO – A shampoo used to treat a condition of the hair and scalp, eg dandruff shampoo.

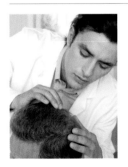

Trichologist – trik-OL-uh-jist – A specialist in hair and scalp disorders, to whom you might refer a client with signs of thinning, weak hair.

Trichology – trik-OL-uh-jee – The science and study of the structure, function and diseases of the human hair and scalp. The clinical branch deals with the diagnosis and treatment of diseases and disorders of human hair and scalp.

Trichorrhexis nodosa – trik-uh-REK-siss noh-DOH-suh – Small, split swellings on the hair shaft where the cortex has split. This is caused by harsh physical and/or chemical damage.

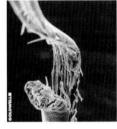
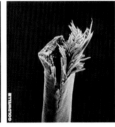

Trichotillomania – TRIK-uh-TIL-uh MAY-nee-uh – This complaint can be associated with some psychiatric illnesses, when areas of hair loss with irregular outlines are caused by the compulsive urge to pull out one's own hair.

Triethanolamine lauryl sulphate – triy-eth-uh-NOL-uh-meen LOR-il SUL-fayt – A soapless detergent – shortened to TLS.

Twist – TWIST – A small section of hair twisted along the length of the head.

Two strand twists

Two strand twists – TOO STRAND TWISTS – Two strands of hair that are twisted to achieve a rope effect.

Two string fly weft – TOO STRING FLY-weft – This is the finest of all weaving and when it is finished, the roots fly away, leaving a neat finish. This is also called a two strand flat weft weave.

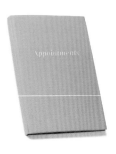

Typical salon reception duties – TIP-ikl SAL-o(ng) or suh-LO(ng) ri-SEP-shuhn DYOO-tiz – These include meeting and greeting clients, checking and making appointments, customer service, and promoting the sale of services and products.

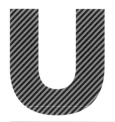

Ultraviolet radiation – UL-truh-VIY-uh-luht ray-dee-AY-shuhn – A way of sterilising tools – remember to turn the tools over, so that each side is sterilised for at least 20 minutes.

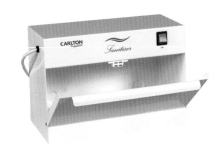

Under-processed – UN-duh-PROH-sesst – Hair that has not been developed to the desired requirements. To rectify this, reapply to the under-processed areas, if the condition allows.

Uneven result – UN-EE-vuhn ri-ZULT – When the service is not the same throughout and does not meet the expected result.

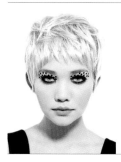

Uniform layer – YOO-ni-form LAY-uh – When all the sections of the hair are the same length from the scalp.

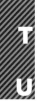

Unique Selling Point (USP) – yoo-NEEK SEL-ing poynt -- YOO-ESS-PEE – Something which makes your product or service stand out from the competition's.

Universal indicator papers – yoo-ni-VUR-suhl IN-di-kay-tuh pay-puhz – A pH indicator that shows if a solution is acid, alkaline or neutral.

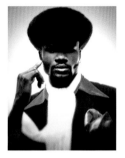

Unusual features – un-YOO-zhuhl FEE-chuhz – Extra care will be needed. These are features that need to be considered when determining the client's requirements. For example, when your client has dimples in the cheeks or chin when facial shaving. You can do this by stretching out the skin to pull out the fold. Other features to take care around are moles or the Adam's apple.

Up-selling – UP-SEL-ing – Recommending a product or service that isn't directly linked to a client's needs and expectations but will enhance their salon or home experience.

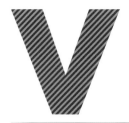

VAT – VAT or VEE-AY-TEE – Stands for value added tax. A VAT-registered business will add VAT to the sale price of most goods and services it offers.

Vegetable dyes – VEJ-tuhbl diyz – The most common vegetable dye is henna; other vegetable colourings are lawsone, camomile, indigo, walnut and quassia.

Vegetable parasite – VEJ-tuhbl PARR-uh-siyt – A fungus.

Vein – VAYN – A blood vessel that carries blood to the heart.

Velcro roller – VEL-kroh ROH-luh – Rollers that stick to the hair and do not need pins.

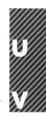

Vellus hair – VEL-uhss HAIR – Fine, downy hair that appears all over our bodies except the palms of the hands and soles of the feet.

Ventilation – ven-ti-LAY-shuhn – The exchanging of air in the salon with fresh air.

Venue – VEN-yoo – The place where a promotional event is held; it might be the local theatre, for instance.

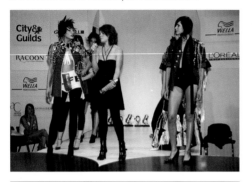

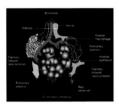

Venule – VEN-yoo-uhl or VEEN-yoo-uhl – A small blood vessel that allows deoxygenated blood to return from the capillaries to the veins.

Vertical roll – VUR-tikl ROHL – A classic dressing that may be worn for a formal event.

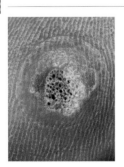

Verruca – vuh-ROO-kuh – A wart on the sole or toes of the foot. The virus attacks the skin through direct contact, generally from walking on moist surfaces, eg showers or swimming pool floors.

Vibrations – viy-BRAY-shuhnz – Moving the fingers on the scalp, which can be stimulating (fast/ firm movement) or soothing (gentle/soft).

Vibro massage – VIY-broh MASS-ahzh or muh-SAHZH – A mechanical device that simulates the manual massage techniques of friction and tapotement. The equipment is like a hairdryer with different attachments that may be used for different areas of the scalp and neck.

Viral infection – VIY-ruhl in-FEK-shuhn – Any type of infection caused by a virus.

Virgin hair – VUR-jin HAIR – Hair that has not had any chemical treatment on it.

Virus – VIY-ruhss – Viruses are too small to be seen with the eye; they can only be seen under a microscope. They are easily spread by coughing, sneezing and touching.

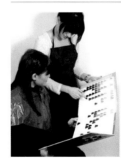

Visual aids – VIZH-yuul AYDZ – Images used during the consultation, for example from style magazines.

Vocational qualifications – vuh-KAY-shuhn-uhl kwol-if-i-KAY-shuhnz – Educational courses that give students the skills they need for a particular profession.

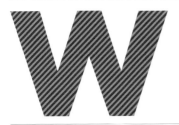

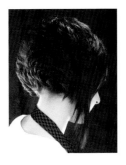

Warm tones – WORM TOHNZ – Yellow, red, copper, brunette and mahogany tones.

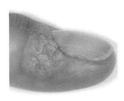

Warts – WORTS (N.B. rhymes with 'ports') – Small growths on the skin caused by a virus.

Waste materials – WAYST muh-TEER-ree-uhlz – Used items that need to be thrown away after the service is completed.

Waste products – WAYST PROD-uhkts – Packaging that may be left over at the end of the service and must be disposed of correctly.

Water pressure – WOR-tuh PRESH-uh – The speed at which the water comes out of the shower head.

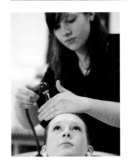

Water temperature – WOR-tuh TEM-pruh-chuh – The heat of the water. This should be checked regularly by asking the client if it feels comfortable.

Wax – WAKS – A product used to create texture and movement in the finished style; it defines and separates individual strands of hair.

Ways of communicating – WAYZ uhv kuh-MYOO-ni-KAY-ting – These include verbal (how you speak) and non-verbal (body language, writing, listening).

Weave perm wind – WEEV PURM WIYND – A technique of weaving a section of hair into two sections before winding to produce movement and root lift.

Weaving frame – WEEV-ing fraym – The right- and left-hand weaving sticks in position on the workbench with the weaving silks affixed.

Weaving silk – WEEV-ing silk – The string of cotton or silk upon which the hair is woven.

Weaving wire

Weaving wire – WEEV-ing wiy-uh – Thin, malleable wire used in the weaving process.

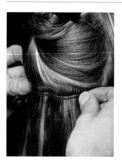

Weft – WEFT – A length of hair woven on silks.

Wefts – WEFTS – Long, continuous strands of pre-coloured hair that create a 'curtain' effect.

When to refer problems – WEN tuh ri-FUR PROB-luhmz – You will need to refer problems to a senior member of staff when the problems are outside your own level of responsibility.

White hair – WIYT HAIR – Also known as canities – hair goes white when it loses its pigmentation, or melanin.

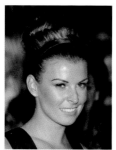

Widow's peak – WID-ohz PEEK – When the hairline goes forward in the centre and back either side.

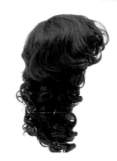

Wig – WIG – Provides full scalp coverage that replaces a natural head of hair.

Winding point to root – WIYND-ing POYNT tuh ROOT – The hair is wound starting from the points (ends) of the hair down to the roots.

Winding root to point – WIYND-ing ROOT tuh POYNT – The hair is wound starting from the root, through the mid-length, and finishing with the ends of the hair.

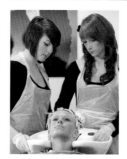

Working co-operatively – WUR-king koh-OP-uh-ri-tiv-lee – Being helpful and supportive of your team.

Working patterns – WUR-king PA-tuhnz – The hours that an employee will work, for example part-time, full-time, or shift work.

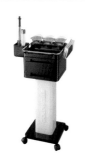

Working safely – WUR-king SAYF-lee – You must make sure you comply with the COSHH regulations (store, handle, use and dispose) when working with colouring products. You must make sure you comply with the health and safety regulations and follow instructions carefully.

Working Time Directive – WUR-king TIYM duh-REK-tiv – Your right not to have to work more than 48 hours a week on average, unless you choose to or work in a sector with its own rules. Your normal working hours should be set out in your employment contract or written statement of employment particulars.

Working Time Regulations – WUR-king TIYM reg-yuh-LAY-shuhnz – This was introduced by the EU (European Union) in order to protect employees from long working hours that would result in a safety hazard due to fatigue.

Working together – WUR-king tuh-GEDH-uh – Being helpful and supportive while making a positive contribution to the team.

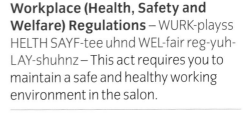

Workplace (Health, Safety and Welfare) Regulations – WURK-playss HELTH SAYF-tee uhnd WEL-fair reg-yuh-LAY-shuhnz – This act requires you to maintain a safe and healthy working environment in the salon.

Workplace policies – WURK-playss POL-iss-iz – Documentation prepared by the employer on the procedures to be followed in the workplace.

Woven effects – WOH-vuhn i-FEKTS – A section of hair is interwoven to obtain a basket weave effect – it can be carried out on a small area, working into other dressing techniques, or over the whole head.

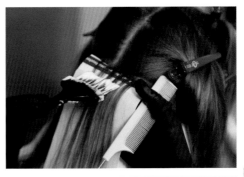

Woven highlights/lowlights – WOH-vuhn HIY-liyts LOH-liyts – A technique using foil or wraps, which is effective in adding multiple colours to hair.

Zygomaticus muscle

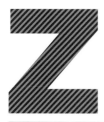

Zygomaticus muscle – ZIY-guh-MAT-ik-uhss MUSSL – The muscle found in the cheekbone that helps to pull the facial expression upward when smiling and laughing.

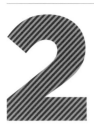

2D surface – too-DEE SUR-fiss –
A design that has been applied to paper.

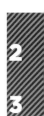

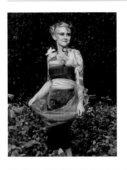

3D surface
– three-DEE SUR-fiss – A design that has been applied to the body or a mannequin.

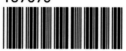